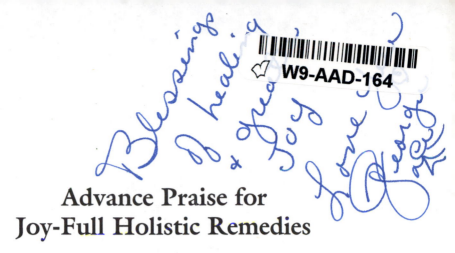

W9-AAD-164

Advance Praise for
Joy-Full Holistic Remedies

"A woman who 'walks her talk' has written of her search for wellness...a journey along many paths to find common sense answers for all ages."

Linda Bedre
President, A New Way
Houston, Texas

"Georgie doesn't know the words 'can't heal.' Her story will encourage and give hope to many who may have temporarily lost their will to go on."

Reverend Jack McGinnis
Freeheart - Addiction Recovery
Desert Hot Springs, California

"Determination helped her heal. This self-help book offers others the gift of life. Physical problems come in many disguises as we push our bodies to their limits."

Vincent Colelli
Heart Transplant Recipient
Texas

JOY-FULL
HOLISTIC REMEDIES

How to Experience
Your Natural Ability
To Heal

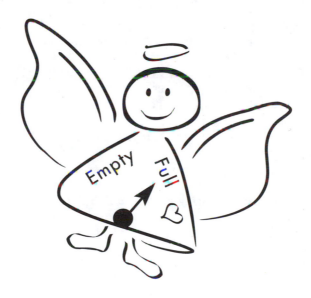

Joy-Full Publishing Company
Houston, Texas

Joy-Full Holistic Remedies
How to Experience Your Natural Ability to Heal
Copyright 1999 by Georgie Holbrook

All rights reserved. This book may not be reproduced in whole or in part by any means, electronic or mechanical, including photocopying, or by any information storage and retrieval system, without written permission from the publisher.

Joy-Full Publishing Company
P.O. Box 591661
Houston, Texas 77259-1661
e-mail: joy_full@earthlink.net
Web page: www.joy-full.com

Editing and layout by Nadine Galinsky
Photographs of author in healthy state (back cover and page 51) provided by Al Ruscelli Photography
Hair styling of author in healthy state (back cover and page 51) by Treva Douglas, Artistic Hair Designer
Cover Design and illustrations on pages 53, 83, and 120 by Gladys Ramirez
Illustrations pages 4 and 76 by Dick Westbrook
Page 20 from *Angel Illustrations* by Marty Noble, 1997 Dover Publications, Inc.

Library of Congress Cataloging-in-Publication Data
Holbrook, Georgie
    Joy-Full Holistic Remedies/Georgie Holbrook.
    ISBN 0-9668742-0-X
    Library of Congress Catalog Card Number: 98-94200

Publisher's Note
    This book represents the author's personal experiences. The information provided in this book is for inspirational and educational purposes only and is specifically not intended as medical or health-related advice. You should check with your physician or health care provider prior to using any remedy or technique discussed in this book.
    This book was printed on acid-free paper.

Joy-Full Holistic Remedies

By God's grace I have been given a second chance. I ask that the gift may now go beyond myself to encourage and offer hope to others.

Allow this book to inspire the love and confidence that comes from using holistic remedies. They are not always easy or fast, but can be rewarding and perhaps even miraculous.

I invite you to read my healing story and, for a brief period, make it your story. Imagine what decisions and actions you would have made. Where would you seek answers? Who is in charge of your health? Do you tend to believe every diagnosis? Do you presently have a diagnosis you have been told you will have for the rest of your life? This book covers prevention and offers holistic solutions for these questions and much more.

This book is exactly what I looked for in my time of need but couldn't find: the details of how someone had healed. I wrote this book knowing how desperate I once was to learn how natural healing takes place and to utilize my own discernment to direct my decisions. My prayer is that my healing journey might be able to shed light on another's path.

When you are finished with this book, be an angel and pass it on to another angel.

I am willing to tell you who I am and share my innermost thoughts in hopes that you can open up to more of your own healing, greatness, and brilliance. You are far greater than your body. Inside of you is a treasure chest with a purpose, holding creativity, joy, laughter, and love wanting to be expressed and experienced. My wish is that you will read my story with reverence for your sacred self, and may God bless you. Remind yourself often that "nothing is impossible with God." Believe always that you can heal!

Georgie

Acknowledgements

I want to dedicate this book to God with thanks for the opportunity to heal holistically, live through a disease, and have the honor of writing this book.

To my parents, Viola and Ralph Nordquist, thanks for sharing life's journey with me. Our strong Scandinavian background has allowed us to withstand the pain of tragic losses and to triumph against all odds.

I want to give special thanks to my husband, William G. "Dub" Holbrook, and his family for helping me to believe in my dreams and follow my heart.

Thanks to Harlan Kidwell, Jr., who came into my life to motivate and inspire me to write my healing story. He blessed not only me but many others who will continually be blessed by the printed words in this book.

Thanks to the late Dr. Maule, herbalist and naturopath from my childhood. You demonstrated in a variety of ways that by creating harmony within the body, the natural system will heal itself. I appreciate his wise spirit and was able to validate what he taught me.

Thanks to Chris Lindsey, artist, poet, and my soul sister. She taught me what inner beauty looks like as it shines outward. I learned about playing as I watched her spirit dance while she painted. Sometimes she blissfully started over with a brand-new creation, much as we can with our lives.

Thanks also to Glory Siller, music minister and chaplain, who invited me to sing and play guitar with her. She helped me excavate a talent that had been dormant for thirty years.

To Nadine Galinsky for her loving inspiration and talent as the editor of this book. With deepest appreciation I give thanks to an angel in human form.

Thanks to Juliann Hemphill and David Williams for their time, talents, and love in critiquing the manuscript. Bless both of you.

Thanks to John D. Huff, M.D., F.A.C.S., my respected mentor and friend for acknowledging alternative medicine and my holistic path. Dr. Huff is truly dedicated to encouraging individuals to utilize their own natural ability to heal.

To Joli Campbell, a young person whose body and mind radiate joy, love, wisdom, and freedom that comes from holistically healing one's past and proudly walking her path.

For consistently inspiring my life and confidence, I give thanks to Treva Douglas, artistic hair designer. Thanks for modeling to the world how one individual can make a difference in others' lives by sharing love, humor, insight, and compassion.

To Carolyn Harper, thanks for the years of dedicating time for building true friendship, allowing both of us to trust exploring deeper thoughts and feelings within ourselves and grow.

I wish to thank my teachers who are many, including my clients, students, and friends who allow me to share in their healing journeys and to learn from them. To my spiritual teachers who have guided me to seek that which is truth for myself, and always to keep an open mind for other people's beliefs and experiences.

Table of Contents

PART ONE
Georgie's Story

This section is my in-depth healing story, including how I made crucial decisions for healing my "incurable," disfiguring disease. I also share my spiritual transformation into the life I now live.

I Am Who I Am

Yet

I Continue To Find More

Of Me

CHAPTER ONE

Disease Doesn't Just Happen!

Who was I before being labeled with a disease? My life certainly looked "Joy-Full" from the outside. I was a business consultant specializing in solving employee, financial, and marketing problems and helping businesses turn a higher profit. Business problems were never "incurable" in my mind. The more difficult the task, the more thrill it gave me. It felt good to know I was needed, and I was rewarded handsomely for my efforts. I had a hefty salary, new cars, homes, wardrobes, material possessions, financial stock, and top-rated credit. I rarely got sick or was inconvenienced by physical pain.

Then suddenly the inevitable, which I had said "would never happen to me," happened as if overnight. I was diagnosed with an incurable and deforming disease. For the next seven years fear, trauma, and uncertainty consumed my life like a raging fire. I felt humiliated to be seen in public, spent all my money and resources in search of a cure, and couldn't see to drive my car or read a book. My life appeared to be over.

For many years I had taken my health for granted. I raced my mind and treated my body like a machine, demanding top performance with little maintenance. I ignored being physically and mentally exhausted. I never turned down a project and became trapped in a compulsive system. Like an alcoholic, work was my "fix," my drug of choice; yet because workaholism is a socially acceptable addiction, I was rewarded and admired for it. I had lost my joy—I was "running on empty." Suddenly, instead of trying to solve my clients' corporate problems, I was forced to focus fully on my own health.

Thank God this was enough of an emergency that I finally took my health seriously, or else I would have continued on my destructive path and probably been driven to an early death of isolation. My God-given talents were wise, intuitive, and extraordinary, yet I had been living a life that, in all honestly, was less than happy.

My routine was rigid and unyielding, consisting of eating, sleeping, and working. There was no time for playing or being in touch with my own personality, my core, or, as some call it, my spirituality. My own body had been trying to tell me something, but I had been too busy to listen. Each day stressed my body like a steady dripping of water onto a piece of concrete—one drip at a time, day after day, unnoticed—eventually wearing a hole large enough that it could not be denied.

Severe allergies were the first sign that my body was rebelling. Then, after five months of allergy shots, the first noticeable symptoms appeared. The skin on my face became very dry and turned bright red. My family physicians agreed the dryness and redness were the result of something I was eating, my hair spray, or my toothpaste. For the next couple of years they treated my condition accordingly. They kept looking for causes in the physical things I was doing or ingesting.

Two years later, with still no results, I met with a skin cancer doctor. He took blood samples and diagnosed me with rosacea, an incurable and disfiguring disease consisting of a chronic fiery red coloration caused by dilation of capillaries, and the appearance of pimples and boils.

I not only got a second opinion, but several other opinions. Giving me little hope, the doctors explained that the disease results in the irreversible deformation of the faces of middle-aged and elderly persons, and

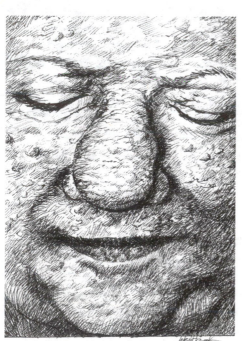

Artist's rendering of face with rosacea

that it is more common in women then in men. Most often this deformation includes an irregular thickening of the skin, which forms knob-like lumps on the face and an enlarged nose; doctors declared that my face would deform in the third year. The disease can also affect the eyes, resulting in a mild to severe decrease in vision.

My future was considered predetermined. Most of the doctors recommended hospitalization. One doctor even called me at home, insisting that I go to the hospital. They wanted to medicate me and then let the disease run its bleak course. In my stubbornness I would not surrender to the doctors' recommendations.

4

I trusted my own judgment and continued to seek answers, knowing that healing was possible.

As time went by, my face became a brighter red, raw, and covered with boils. The embarrassment of being a female in midlife with a face that looked like it had been in a fire caused me deep emotional pain. I dreaded being seen in public but taught myself how to act callused to others' comments when I was. Innocent children screamed with fear when they saw me in the supermarket or on the sidewalk, thinking they had seen a monster. Their honesty left deep, long-lasting scars on my psyche. Adults were no more helpful with their constant questions of, "How did it happen?" "What kind of disease do you have?" "What happened to you!!" They bombarded me with remedies from helpful to ridiculous, day after day and year after year. My wounded spirit felt very helpless, and I suffered enormous shame about my appearance.

During the first few years of my disease, I assumed that all physicians had detailed information about human physiology, and I expected them to know how a healthy cell changes to become unhealthy or, in my case, how healthy facial skin turns red and develops boils. No matter how often I asked, however, I couldn't get this core information.

But I never gave up hope. "What caused this disease to develop?" I kept asking, wanting a doctor to explain how my immune system works and how my body heals. I searched diligently for doctors and specialists who might lead me to the answers I was seeking. I asked each doctor I contacted for the names of other doctors who might have more information. I contacted these people by phone, in person, or by mail. I found centers that specialized in rare diseases, but none specialized in rosacea. Some doctors suggested new drugs on the market that offered a possibility, but they really were only wild guesses. Most doctors were not knowledgeable or interested in dietary issues, so there was little guidance about what foods, if any, to avoid or consume. There certainly was no concern expressed for how this diagnosis affected me emotionally.

The only consistent recommendations I received were drugs, topical creams, and hospitalization. Even then, the doctors indicated this course of treatment would be experimental with no real guarantees or knowledge of potentially dangerous side effects. Many of the doctors did not agree with each other about the types of drugs to use. Some offered me free samples of drugs to try, but I decided the real price was too expensive. I believed that once I was drugged, I would be out of control and I would no longer be able to make important decisions about my life. In my belief system, this would be just copping out and hoping the rosacea would go away. I was also afraid of how these drugs would affect my

5

organs, such as the liver and kidneys, which appeared to be functioning normally.

I prayed daily not to deform as badly as the pictures I was shown, but I was convinced I would deform. I was driven by two internal voices: One was the business consultant who demanded, "Don't tell me I can't heal!" I couldn't even comprehend the thought of not getting well. Business problems were never unsolvable, and certainly not forever. The other voice was of the scared child who wanted to cry and plead, "Please don't tell me I can't heal."

Later I met two other people with rosacea. One who was on cortisone was now scarred for life, her facial skin twisted with lesions the size of quarters. The other was in a nursing home because her entire face was now disfigured and she couldn't stand the pain of being seen in public. After meeting them, I was certain I would never, ever be strong enough to live the rest of my life looking so ugly and grotesque, and losing any part of my eyesight. After this I would not allow my mind ever to consider what I would do if the worst did happen. I built a solid wall in my mind and never asked myself the "what if" questions.

I had a lot invested in the direction I was choosing, really stepping out and not following what "they" told me. I knew I was walking a strange path, feeling alone yet determined that any problem had to have a solution. In the meantime weeks were passing, and my condition wasn't waiting for me to get educated.

My search for answers included health food stores, libraries, health agencies, holistic healers, healed people, books, healing magazines, and massage therapy. I also asked for referrals at many of these places and diligently investigated each lead.

I tried fasting from nine to fourteen days in hopes of resting my organs and assisting my immune system to function more effectively. Each time I observed how this fasting affected my body. I learned to feel the difference between a fruit and vegetable juice diet. I learned which foods made me feel good and which made me feel sluggish, which foods gave me indigestion, and which foods resulted in aches and pains. I had professional colonics to clean my colon. I learned to give myself an enema so that I could keep my colon cleaned of toxins. I cautiously applied various natural ointments and creams to my face, but even aloe vera felt like acid. I studied with every natural healer I could find and tried anything that made sense and even some suggestions that seemed far-fetched. Following the Bible's promise, "Seek and ye shall find," I was not just seeking, but seeking desperately.

6

After about three years I met a doctor's wife who convinced me that her 75-year-old husband, a dermatologist specializing in skin diseases, could help me. She was convincing, so I traveled a long distance to meet with him.

I remember having such high hopes of getting answers from him. He was very gentle, but after examining me said that in thirty-five years of practice he had never seen a case of this disease that didn't result in deformation. He had no suggestions or recommendations. I felt like a hot-air balloon filled with faith and hope that was instantly punctured and ripped open, tumbling emotionally down, frayed and torn into nervous threads from one more disappointing lead.

I gathered myself up and I did the only thing I knew how: I pushed on. I wondered how long it would be before I began to deform. A friend told me much later that I **had** begun to deform, but I did not admit it to myself, and of course, no one pointed that fact out to me. If I had realized my true state, I might have given up.

Later that year, in the extreme heat of the summer, I flew from North Carolina to Alabama. I checked into a holistic medical center located on 25 acres of beautiful rolling hills and forest and began three weeks of evaluations. The five medical doctors there used a program consisting of patient education, lifestyle evaluation, medical exams, and natural treatments and remedies. This center attracted people from all over the world with major health problems—cancer, diabetes, coronary disease, and arthritis, among others. I was very impressed by the results the patients were experiencing and determined that body chemistry and the natural harmony of our bodies must be similar. Seeing these similarities, I wondered why our world made healing so complicated. Would I ever uncover the necessary information to see healing in my life?

This center sent people into the country to find God, peace of mind, and healing in nature. It was a haven of beauty and holistic medicine. Part of the therapy included exercise, sunshine, rest, gardening, cooking classes, herbs, and water therapy. Gathering together daily to pray for each other, the patients had created an environment that encouraged healing by bringing the body back into a more natural state of peacefulness and harmony.

My three-week regimen included a walking program, a diet consisting of homegrown fresh fruits and vegetables, juices, and homemade breads, and large quantities of garlic, known to help cleanse the blood. I had a private room, and the staff did everything possible to see that I was comfortable. I noticed the treatments didn't hurt me physically or make me feel bad. I might have felt a little weak at times, but I recovered quickly.

I had hydrotherapy (water treatments) five to six days a week. I was placed in a steam chamber, and my temperature was raised to 104 degrees. Although I lost so much weight by sweating that I could eventually count my ribs, my facial skin never showed any signs of moisture or opening up to breathe.

After three weeks my face was even more raw and a much brighter red. The doctors met with me and said they had no answers. Their observation was that every layer of skin on my face was like a scar. I asked about having my face sanded to attract healing from deeper layers, but they doubted this was possible in my case, because a scar is a scar in the deep inner skin also.

Although the people at this center did not offer emotionally supportive therapy, only physical treatments and spiritual practices, I detected that they were on to something significant in what they did offer. I had witnessed people with chronic problems healing at this same center and had read testimonies from others. I also felt more accepted there than out in the world. I felt ugly, in the way I suspect lepers do. I wanted to find a safe place to live away from the stress of being judged bad, incurable, or diseased. I went home and convinced my husband that I wanted to go back and live at this center to study, work, and be a patient.

Between the cost of my husband's education (he had received his master of divinity degree) and my frantic search for my health, funds were not available for a move across the country. I didn't feel that I had any choice, though, so we proceeded to sell all our valuables, including treasured pieces of jewelry from my business days. Everything was sold, stripping us down to bare necessities. We knew we would have to work once we arrived at the health facility. For me, the stress of work wasn't in my best interest as a patient, but it was a risk I was willing to take.

Once we arrived and got settled at the center, my schooling began. I was fascinated by the results these people were getting. I studied with both the staff and patients, looking for any clues to my own perplexing problem. The entire experience was very educational, but frustrating as well. After two years of treatment I had gotten progressively worse, losing nearly eighty percent of my eyesight. The first stage of deforming was apparent. When my husband received a ministerial opportunity in Oregon, we sadly moved on.

From what I had experienced up until now, I came to the conclusion that, in order to heal, we must consider our entire lifestyle. A balance is necessary for healing to take place, and nutrition plays a major part because we become what we eat. Exercise, rest, sunshine, and getting out in nature are all basic ingredients for healing.

All of this time, though, I never addressed the issue of what I was feeling, nor did anyone else. No one was sensitive enough to notice or ask the painful questions: "How do you deal emotionally with having people stare at you like you are turning their stomachs?" or, "How does it feel to be diseased, knowing that deforming could begin any day?" "Do you consider suicide?" "Are you angry?" "How do you cope with the enormous grief of losing your eyesight and appearance?" "How does it feel to continue to research and try over and over again, yet be given no real hope?" "How does it feel to lance boils every day with a sterile needle and watch your facial skin become more and more leathery?" "Do you need a friend to confide in?" No one came to me with an open heart asking how I felt about living with this dreadful ordeal. I felt isolated and terrorized. My emotions froze deep inside of me. I disassociated from myself and those around me, just trying to survive.

How did my husband respond to my having a disease? I suspect he was very scared, and in his fear separated emotionally from my desperate attempts to get help. He did the best he knew how. He could see I was hurting but couldn't feel or empathize with my pain.

Both of us continued in workaholic fashion not to talk about the tragedy that was taking place. The doctors had predicted, and therefore we expected, permanent deforming to happen any day after the second year. On occasion my husband would sit across the table from me while eating and look at my face. He would say things like, "I think your nose is starting to enlarge," or "I'm noticing your face getting worse." I would panic and run into the bathroom to check. Interestingly, I never could see the changes he pointed out. Either I was in denial or just not convinced.

There were occasions when he showed sympathy. Once he went with me to a doctor's office and helped two nurses hold me down on a table while the doctor surgically removed an infected, large, hard boil the size of a pea from my eyelid. He responded when I needed help, but most of the time I kept my thoughts, feelings, and needs to myself.

Our health insurance would have paid for my complete hospitalization, and my husband tended to side with the doctors to have me go that route. From his perspective it appeared to be the most economical and medically wise course to take. The doctors' recommendations were persuasive, but I was never convinced. Looking back, I realize it took a lot of courage to stand by my truth and be willing to put my money where my heart was.

Up until now, mostly unknown to me, only God and the angels kept me from destroying myself as I continually sought help. I didn't have much faith in God. Instead I felt separated from God and frustrated that the answers were so slow in coming. I was anointed and prayed over for healing many times, but the requests appeared to go unnoticed. By this time I was exhausted from trying so hard to get results, but doors did open and I continued to walk through them as if God was leading me by the hand.

I was led next to a dermatology and skin specialist conference where more than 150 doctors gathered to share information about rare skin diseases. I had the dubious honor of being selected as one of their case studies. Again, I was very hopeful about finding the answers I had been looking for. I felt grateful and positive.

Then came the letdown. I had gone way beyond the three-year time frame when deforming normally took place. The doctors wanted to know what I was doing differently, because I was so much better off than most patients they had seen with this disease were. The roles were reversed. I was giving them answers. I didn't learn anything except that they were very impressed with the results I was getting. I knew from their comments that what I had learned to do for myself was having a positive impact.

After six years of holistic remedies and the advice of countless medical experts, I still had not given up hope, but disappointments had left me feeling defeated over and over again. I felt angry, sad, lonely, helpless, and beaten down by the medical system. Life was very difficult, almost impossible to comprehend, and nearly unbearable. Where was God? Was God really going to let me deform and become nearly blind or even lose my eyesight because I couldn't find in the world what my heart knew was always possible: a solution? **Was it pointless to fight against such devastating odds?**

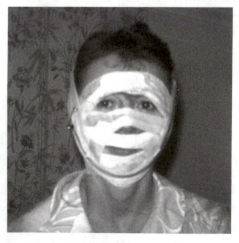

CHAPTER TWO

The Solution Isn't Always Obvious

Living with rosacea for all those years caused deep emotional pain. It would take many more years to get in touch with and heal the depths of the terror and devastation I had experienced. In order to be able to tolerate the intensity of this disease, I buried the memories deep within my body where I could not access them, as in a reserve bank account. This gave me the emotional stability and courage to keep persevering.

All along, my body had been prepared through nutrition for healing. Six years into my journey I went on garlic therapy to a greater extent than I had before. I ate raw and streamed garlic for three meals a day. It wasn't pleasant, but it wasn't unbearable either. I don't know what my body smelled like, but I knew I had to keep trying, never giving up.

After about four months of garlic therapy, I woke up with my same fire-red face all broken out with boils, but this day was different. My face was so swollen I could barely open my mouth or eyes. My first thought was that the deforming had started. Fear grabbed my guts.

Sometime later that day, I realized that fear was sending me internally into hysterics. I switched my mind-set and affirmed, "I'm healing! Yes, I'm healing!" over and over the rest of the day. My mind began to calm my fears and switch my thinking from dreadful, scary thoughts to, "This could actually be what I've been praying for." The possibility of its being, even in a small way, a positive sign was a welcome surprise.

Much later that day the swelling started going down, and very thin pieces of skin the size of quarters started rolling off. It was like a bad case of sunburn peeling, but worse. It lasted two days and never happened again. My face actually didn't look any different than before, but I knew something significant had happened. My facial skin had given me a sign that it was still alive. I credited the garlic for this change and continued the daily routine for another three months before gradually tapering off.

Even with this encouragement, I was still determined to find answers about the healing process. I was invited to another holistic health conference in California, where medical doctors presented new insights on preventing cancer, coronary disease, stroke, and health problems in

11

general. They set up living quarters at the center so patients could stay while going through diet, exercise, education, and lifestyle changes. I was there as a student and patient eager to learn.

I was assigned to Dr. Lee, a Korean medical doctor, for my physical exam. This man was different from all the other doctors I had seen. Immediately I knew I had met a real friend who wanted to help me. He prayed with me and was extremely observant of my body language and the details of my condition.

Dr. Lee came to the United States to become a doctor because he wanted to understand how healing takes place and how the immune system gets strengthened to prevent illness and disease. He was fortunate to have grown up with natural healers as his mentors. They saw the human body as a self-healing system and believed that disease and illness were the body's way of crying out for help to get back to a natural state of health and vitality.

Dr. Lee was informed in medical school that this was not part of the curriculum, but he could learn about medications and surgery in relationship to physical problems and ailments. After completing his formal training, he then began to conduct his own intensive studies on the immune system and healing.

Up until this time I had perceived doctors as almost godlike. They presumably had so much more education than I did about healing and the human body. Now, six years later, I was remarkably self-educated and determined to couple my knowledge with someone else's to reach a solution. This was the doctor I had been searching for, who lived what he believed and treated me with respect and reverence. He encouraged me to tell him in detail the methods I had tried.

Dr. Lee went through my medical file and noticed the allergy vaccine I had taken before the onset of rosacea. He said he had studied this vaccine, and it was known to have side effects. He then gave me his interpretation of what had happened to me. He explained that when people drive themselves in life or the corporate fast track for years, they diminish their ability to ward off illness and disease. This lowered immunity becomes even worse with allergy vaccines. Apparently I had run myself down so that my own inherent healing abilities could no longer function properly.

After observing me and listening to my internal body sounds, Dr. Lee remarked that with my clothes on, I looked fairly normal with the exception of my face. However, this appearance was deceiving. He noted that my body temperature was uneven to his touch. My hands and feet were chilled. The backs of my arms were a different temperature from the rest of my arms, and there were similar temperature variations all over my body.

In addition to these observations, my insides felt like they had a continual nervous shiver, and I had a tight knot-like feeling in my stomach. I constantly had a pain in my chest. My body temperature would rise one to two degrees instantly under any stressful situation, and my face would flush an even brighter red. I felt very fragile, frail, and vulnerable.

Dr. Lee picked up on the quivering I was feeling inside. He actually could get quiet enough to feel the functions of my internal systems and sense the difference between normal and abnormal motion. He said the constant turmoil of people being in an emergency situation for so long sets up a perpetual, extreme negative condition that stresses all body systems. My natural biological rhythms were no longer in harmony, so vital energy had decreased.

Put plainly, fear was eating away my life. The awful dread of imminent, permanent deforming was killing me. For the first time, someone was acknowledging my fear and exploring what it was doing to my physical condition. Dr. Lee proved to me by his insight that my body was overcompensating and running on nervous energy rather than in a peaceful balance. He explained that the best nutrition fed to a body in trauma helps only in a limited way, because stress and fear destroy the benefits.

I had become what I thought about most—worry and fear—and my mind fed my body the same messages. Emotional pain was destroying my body, face, and eyes. My internal body turmoil was a cry for help.

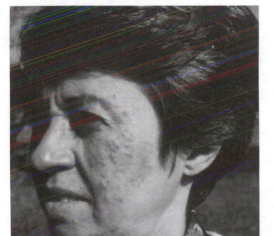

Dr. Lee gently proceeded by explaining that my emotional stability played a major part in my health and healing. People who are happy and peaceful have a body chemistry that reflects their lifestyle. They have figured out ways to express their emotions to stay in a healthy balance. Being unhappy, traumatized, fearful, and worried restricts the system and sets up an artificial pattern for just coping with life. But the good news was that the dynamo of the human body was always ready and willing to heal. The only reason healing wouldn't be possible would be if the damage had gone too far.

I remember his formula: "A healthy cell is a happy cell!" I hadn't experienced happiness or healthy fun for so many years, I had almost forgotten they were possible. I had created so many restrictions in my life that I didn't have a life.

He applauded all my efforts, but said the bottom line was that my whole body chemistry was out of harmony. This disease wasn't just on my face! That's where all the focus had been up until now. How could I heal the symptoms when I hadn't looked at other causes of my disability?

Dr. Lee said he didn't have any guarantee that I would ever heal, but said I should seek a state of internal peace. It made sense! Bring the body back into harmony. Move out of fear. Seek joy. At this time those words felt very foreign, but I was a willing, eager student. All I needed was information and a direction.

He was my first sign of hope and the first one to give me answers that made sense to me. He told me about the immune system and how it works, but the most important thing was that I could neither heal nor have a meaningful life living in a body filled with fear. He said I must take my attention off the effects on my face and focus on the possible cause of my own emotional pain. All those doctors, six to ten a year for many years, ugly pictures, and verbal pronouncements about my condition had taken their toll. I knew I must discover this peace within, whatever the price.

A core belief I held up until this time was that I had a disease, so therefore *I* must be diseased. When I looked in the mirror, I looked ugly, so therefore *I* must be ugly. I felt unlovable and shameful for my own lack of self-love. Diet and nutrition had been my only hopes of healing. I had spent hours preparing a natural diet of fresh fruits, vegetables, nuts, grains, beans, and juices, always trying to improve my efforts. My reasoning was that if I could feed my body well enough, I stood a better chance of healing. My body was becoming what I was feeding it. What I lacked was the understanding of what to feed my mind and spirit.

After returning to Oregon, I enrolled in a four-hour, once-a-week stress class at a local hospital. There were about ten people in this class. I was terrified to be seen by others. I wanted information, but at the same time I wanted to hide. I truly looked like I had been burned. I was so scared of being asked to talk that I really didn't hear anything the teacher said.

I was then led to an organization that did personal effectiveness training, presenting study and experiential workshops on how fear, abuse, childhood trauma, addictions, and dysfunctions interrelate with our minds, emotions, and bodies. Their goal was to get people to have healthier bodies, rewarding relationships, financial stability, and perhaps even new careers. This was not a medical facility, but local counselors and trainers who saw a need and started a business of helping lay people and executives find answers. The facilitators were people who had gone through their own hardship and pain, and now wanted to share what they were learning about mental and emotional health with others.

I met with a counselor and gave her all the reasons I didn't feel strong enough to go into a two-week workshop with eighty people. I felt I would die exposed to so many strangers, and I was afraid of placing myself under any more stress. I felt very close to the breaking point. Perhaps I felt I would lose my mind or end my life. It was very scary. The counselors decided that one of them would sit beside me for the first day or two to support me if I needed it.

This was my first emotional-therapy or mental-health group. Eighty class members shared their own devastating stories. For the first time I was with people who were willing to relate to me rather than interrogate me. They helped me believe that I could breathe a little easier and stop trying to act so brave. I started to relax ever so slightly. I felt safe with these people even though I didn't mingle much. I noticed within the first few hours of being around emotionally honest folks that it was feeding my soul. I not only felt calmer, but my face did also. I knew in my heart that I was on to something significant and that my emotional state of well-being would play an important part in my healing.

When I started the class, I was extremely shut down, both emotionally and physically. My feelings were not available to me in any form that I could translate. I just felt numbed out, exhausted, sad, and ugly. I was very afraid and quiet. I never volunteered to talk, but secretly the pain I felt screamed inside of me, ready any moment to erupt into talking deliriously. I controlled myself, not speaking unless called on directly, and then my words were brief and came out only with others coaching me.

I watched others heal and, like osmosis, I began to heal through them. What I couldn't express, they expressed. Some yelled in anger in order to release their emotions from being abused or treated unfairly, and their yells penetrated my walls of self-made armor and helped me release my own internal cry for help. I received an incredible amount of reassurance when I realized that my situation was not that different from that of the others.

I had lived for some six years theorizing about having a disease, without having knowledge of the impact of emotional trauma and emotional pain. This was no less significant than a combat veteran who was now supposed to act like nothing happened during the war. This group started to help me heal my deep inner scars.

I witnessed many healing episodes that further convinced me I had discovered answers to my search. One woman who had used a cane for years was soon walking without one. People who were on insulin for diabetes suddenly didn't require as much as before. Others who had been taking allergy drugs began to take less. One person with asthma began to have less difficulty breathing. People gave up cigarettes and began to smell fresh air again. People who had acted out sexually and violated their bodies began to talk openly about it. They began to heal that angry part of themselves. People changed physically, looking softer and less intense. They became more spontaneous, even to the point of dancing.

We all were being challenged to look at our beliefs and patterns of behavior and to effect change. We each in our own way made a statement to our world that we were committed to our own growth and freedom from bondage.

I had to acknowledge that my life until now was void of any joy. I'll always remember my very first day. We were asked to list all the people, places, things, and beliefs we enjoyed, and those we didn't. My list consisted of ninety-five percent dislikes, including my religion. These were my thoughts:

***

Religion had been the pivotal point around which everything else in my life centered. Now church was on my list of high-stress events I could no longer cope with. My church obligations appeared impossible to decline. I felt as if I was committed to them for life, because my husband was a minister.

Reflecting back on his years in seminary, I remember being taught not to share our emotions or personal life with the congregation. Instead we were to show an unreal but ideal picture of a perfect lifestyle. I realized I was very lonely, isolated emotionally, and even desperate for friends with whom I could share my feelings.

My list of dislikes also included some rigid church people who secretly would give me scripture trying to prove to me that disease was not of God. They judged me unjustly, saying, "If you were walking with God, you would be healed." "If only you had enough faith, God would heal you." "There must be something you did in the past that was bad and you are being punished." "You need to ask forgiveness." I was honestly baffled by this one. I didn't have a clue what to ask forgiveness for. The most ridiculous comment was, "This is the cross you have to bear as a witness for being able to suffer for the Lord."

After awhile I started feeling somewhat crazy, judged by those who thought their interpretation of God's word was gospel, and that they were God's only righteous helpers. Being very sick, I also started thinking negative thoughts and pondering if perhaps I actually was the condemned person they declared me to be.

On several occasions, some medical doctors in our church made fun of me in front of others for choosing my holistic route. In their own arrogance of playing God, they chose to judge my path, rather than having compassion for a person in transformation.

***

After completing the list of likes and dislikes, I began to make major changes in my lifestyle. Three months later, another workshop became available with the same organization. Seventy people attended, and the facilitator asked the big question: "How many of you have been diagnosed in the past with chronic symptoms, diseases, or ailments, and were told you would have them the rest of your lives?" I lost count of the raised hands. "What types of diagnoses?" People responded with diabetes, blood pressure, nervous disorders, memory-loss, arthritis, cancer, and others. I responded with rosacea.

I thought, "What is this all about?" We were then asked to identify the first symptoms; mine were allergies. Then we were asked, "What happened three to six months prior to the first symptoms? Did something tragic happen, such as the death of a significant friend or family member, divorce, job loss, emotional or physical abuse, etc.?" They had determined the importance of identifying the traumatic event and linking it to our symptoms and diagnoses. We were told that if we could release the trauma from our minds and body that took place during the intensity of the event, our diagnoses, "our incurables" would possibly go away or lessen. I thought, "This is insightful, if someone has really discovered this to be true!"

We were given time to write and relive those months prior to our diagnoses. What happened next became very revealing to me. I began writing about the twelve months prior to my first allergy symptoms, before the disease was identified. Following is a summary of what I learned:

***

17

I remembered going to the doctor for aches in the joints of my hands, elbows, neck, and shoulders and being told they couldn't find anything wrong with me. The aches were blamed on stress. In my heart, I knew my fast-paced life was beginning to catch up with me. I was in denial about how unhappy I was.

About a month later, my husband decided that what he wanted more than anything else was to get his masters degree in divinity, and to become a minister. He was in the corporate world but had previously, before I had met him, been in the ministry. In the business world I had always considered myself on a mission, striving to make a positive difference in life, so ministry didn't seem to be any different. I imagined it to be a slower, more loving way to share my talents with others.

I had always responded to life automatically saying "yes," without really looking at the demands on me. In a weak moment, without considering the consequences, I agreed to find one of my high-paying corporate jobs and cover all our financial expenses. Decisions were made quickly, and he enrolled in a two-year seminary program.

We moved to Michigan for the start of a new career that promised, hopefully, to be fulfilling for both of us. Seminary graduate school had a two-year program for those students who didn't have to work and a four-year program for those who did. We were told by school officials that this new life was built on trust and having faith in God to supply all our needs.

Upon arriving and getting settled I soon discovered there were no large corporations, only farming and small industry. I ended up working two jobs six days a week. I had to make enough money to cover our monthly expenses, his tuition, and child support payments for his two children.

Exactly three months from the start of his first ministerial class, I developed all types of symptoms; shortness of breath, pains in my stomach, insomnia, headaches, and constant worry about the load I was carrying. I called a family meeting and shared my overwhelming feelings with him. I asked, "Would you be willing to get part-time work to help us out?"

"It's only two years," he replied. "You only need to do it for two years, then we'll be together." His heart was set on graduating and getting his first church assignment. He had been out of school for a number of years and it was all he could do to keep up with his studies. I tried to reason with him, but he refused to change or compromise.

My desperate need was left unheard, and I felt not respected as a human, let alone his wife. I felt outraged and trapped, and it felt as though

I would die if I had to keep pushing so hard; yet the bills continued to come in. I didn't think or feel I had any choice but to serve. I was the "glorified seminarian's wife," and my first assignment in that role was too much to ask of me, and for sure my body and health. I was reminded from my culture that I should "stand by my man," but I felt personally violated. With the weight of the world bearing down on my shoulders, I felt as though I had been handed a death sentence.

Within days I developed severe allergies, sneezing almost nonstop. I had too big a responsibility to get sick, so I proceeded to get allergy shots, hoping the problem would go away! As I looked back, I saw that this symbolized how I, too, wanted to "go away!" For the next five months, I visited the allergy doctor twice a week for shots, and they appeared to work. The symptoms went away. Or did they? At this point my face started breaking out with pimples and turning red.

I did the only thing I knew how to do—I numbed out. I worked beyond the point of exhaustion for the next two years, like an iron soldier. Six months before my husband completed his seminary studies, I was diagnosed with rosacea.

I do have some wonderful memories mixed in with the hard parts from this time in my life. It was almost like taking a trip around the world. I got to meet people from many different cultures and was introduced to their clothing, foods, music, education, and beliefs, and viewed pictures of their homelands. I was very impressed and will treasure this experience the rest of my life.

***

Now, seven years later the disease was recognized for what it was, and over time layers upon layers of pain were being heard, released and healed with gratitude, love, and thanksgiving. This workshop and organization was so appropriate for me at this time in my life. It was obvious to me that what they were sharing was "truth;" my health had improved noticeably every week from the day I first attended their classes. My face was now showing miraculous signs of healing, and my eyesight was getting better. I couldn't dispute their philosophy. I reminded myself, though, that I had taken many steps towards improving my general health before ever hearing about this organization; it is important to recognize this fact. For me, there was no quick fix!

Then our class was given further insights. We were told that throughout our experiences, if we could have had someone hold us, to allow our innermost being to rest, to allow us to cry and talk, and to be listened to without having our feelings minimized, we would have experienced a very different outcome; in fact, our symptoms may not have had to develop into our diagnoses.

They were right! This part had been missing for me. I remember longing to be held, listened to, and encouraged to cry, but no one offered and I was too sick to ask. At times I had fantasized living in the forest where I knew I would be comforted, accepted, safe, and could cry, moan, wail, rest, and be perfectly still. This forest would be similar to the forest where I grew up as a child.

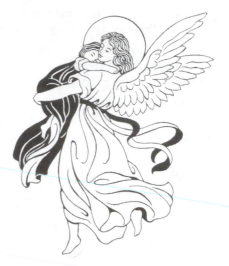

The class was a time of awakening, for I had become buried alive in stress, disease, diet, emotional pain, self-betrayal, fear, false religion, and loneliness. I had to let go of what wasn't working and create a new life for myself. I remember what a pleasant thought that was. It felt like the most freeing solution I had ever heard. I started to remove those things I didn't like, and I started to fill my life with things I could "face" and "see" with joy and gratitude. With every direction for healing I had taken over the last seven years, I had gone at it with all my heart and changed, sometimes 180 degrees in a new direction. This was one of those times. Overnight I cleaned house and didn't leave anything unnoticed. My life felt a little void for a period of time, but I welcomed with celebration the refreshing changes. My superwoman business mentality rescued me as I set up boundaries of what I would and would not do.

I started on a new path of healing. I cried and grieved my experiences in group and individual emotional therapy. I refocused and determined what I wanted in my new life. I learned ways to love and appreciate Georgie. Therapists and therapy support groups were very nurturing, and I discovered that my experience wasn't that much different than others, wounded people willing to ask for help and healing.

Interestingly, when I needed therapy, I began to trust that as I took care of myself, money would be available. Many times I received pleasant surprises; money came in, sometimes on the exact day it was needed.

CHAPTER THREE

A New Life Revealed

Dr. Lee had said to find peace within, a remedy that sounds fairly easy, and maybe even free of charge. I had finished months of emotional therapy and had made many changes, but how could I achieve the degree of inner peace he recommended? What did that look and feel like? I was ready for my next assignment, and my next teacher appeared.

By this time I was promoting an eight-week workshop on making lifestyle changes to prevent illness and disease, a program approved by many hospitals and doctors. My minister husband gave the lectures, and I did all the coordinating. I did phone sales and marketing, still avoiding direct contact with strangers because my face, although showing signs of improvement, was still very red.

We were asked to do a health program at a church, so I went to meet with the minister, Reverend Ingram. He radiated joy and love without saying a word. His eyes danced with an excitement for life. They were clear, almost translucent. The essence and presence of what I had imagined a "holy man" would look like, he seemed to embody the spirit of the Christ. I was spellbound by meeting a real master teacher. The Bible says, "You will know them by their fruits." His internal fruits radiated like a beacon, beckoning me to notice his internal light.

Instantly something inside of me said, "This is what peace must look like in a human body." My soul hungered to be fed and spirit filled. I knew spirituality meant finding peace in my soul. Unreleased anger and fear were disturbances of my heart and great obstacles to the presence of a spirit within me. In more than four decades I had never met anyone with his attributes. He had discovered internal peace and a connection with his Creator. I felt like he was elderly, yet he hadn't aged. My mind raced with excitement. I wondered: was it possible for all children created to be taught through these inherent attributes to live more abundantly? I immediately decided I wanted to experience for myself the qualities he radiated. We conducted the health program, but I was led to this church for my own spiritual healing.

This church was open to all religions and cultures. It was Christian-based, but with the focus on educating people in scientific principles about the universe and how our God-given minds and bodies operate. Principles as accurate as gravity and mathematics were taught, along with how to apply the perfection of God in daily lives, eliminating guesswork and confusion. They taught that God is as near as getting quiet and listening for the "still small voice" that gives reliable direction.

I became a student of this minister. He explained to me that he didn't believe that God was a God of punishment, or that an evil force or Satan had been out to get me. But he did believe that each pain and illness has its own distinct cry or complaint, and that the universe and all of creation operate on perfection and principles that I could prove. If I violated these principles I would get signals that, if I ignored them, would increase or get worse.

He showed me that stuffed emotions, unexpressed and unacknowledged, would manifest in the body as "art forms" or "parables." These forms take on an appearance that cause minor to great discomfort, even boils on the face and closing off the circulation of every layer of skin.

The art form expressed by the body would also hold the answers. If it was in the eyes, it was about "not liking what I was seeing in my own life." If it was my heart, it would be tied into love and security. The breast would be about nurturing, and lungs about sadness or grieving. He said I could find books available for me to study this phenomenon.

I was intrigued. Was God actually working individually with us, if only we were listening to our body language? Did God create children in God's image, equipped inherently with an internal guidance system that, if followed, would be very rewarding and bring tremendous fulfillment? Could this guidance system take the doubt out of living and end empty, disconnected feelings? Why would God create a precious child without direct internal communications? God didn't, I realized; I had drifted far away from my own guidance system, but was being reconnected fast.

I was trying to be open and learn. This was Reverend Ingram's truth, but was it mine? I had become a tough student for God, because I was very cautious. "Prove it to me. I'm open and receptive to learning a better way." Resisting didn't seem helpful, so I determined I would take what fit and leave the rest. I knew that whatever felt uncomfortable or foreign to me might have more meaning later on, so I stayed open to concepts I couldn't immediately adapt to my belief system.

I had created a far-off God from some invisible space I called heaven. Reverend Ingram suggested that I re-evaluate my beliefs. What I believed about God was also what I believed about myself, creating distance from myself. Suddenly I was open to a new world of thinking that I knew was truth for me.

Reverend Ingram taught me principles I could apply in my daily life. He said if God was anywhere, God was everywhere, equally present. "You mean God was also with me through that disease when I felt so separated?" I asked. Yes, it was like God was in a helicopter, guiding my every step.

Speculating, Reverend Ingram asked me, "Would it be worth going through the experience you had, if in the end you could become instrumental in world healing?"

My immediate response without one doubt was, "Of course!" I felt like Jesus was standing next to me and reminding me of his own demonstration through death, saying life is meant to bring us to our own resurrection story.

I felt exhausted and encouraged at the same time. I had been through a war and had been literally brainwashed by others and myself. As long as my mind was convinced I had this dreadful disease, that was all I thought about and studied.

How could I start reprogramming my mind? I learned the principle of using my imagination correctly. Whatever I focus on expands. My brilliant brain will help me create that which I continually imagine. It allows me to think of fearful things or loving, positive things. It aids me in giving me my desires. It had even aided the process of my disease by my being so convinced of its cause. How else would any normal person react to all those pictures of deformed faces and articles of the deforming process and vision loss? The power of the spoken and printed word stunned me.

Amazed by the power of this principle, my confusion began melting away. I had been misusing my own imagination and programming my body based on fear. I opened my life to gratitude for the enormous healing and insight I was experiencing. I would now continue to change the messages sent to my body.

I was ready to learn a better way and receive the good from all people. Some of what I was learning really stretched me; it was all challenging, exciting, and rewarding, so I made a decision to stay open to possibilities. I began to realize that I had a unique and special purpose on this planet, and finding that purpose would bring me the most joy and fulfillment. I needed to heal my exhaustion and to rest until those doors opened.

Reverend Ingram said that we are all divinely guided individuals, provided we are open to that guidance. By seeking and experiencing silence I could, over time, connect with the spiritual aspects of myself and find inner peace. He said my innate desires would become obvious as I allowed myself to be guided from my inner harmony and joy, from which flows a powerful hidden energy of healing, spiritual awakening, creativity, and a clear, divine direction for my life. This was a process that I began to apply and trust.

I continued to be led, as my soul was hungry to be filled more with the "holy man" attributes of joy and celebration. With so much to consider and re-evaluate, I felt like a little child, filled with wonder at this new world I was seeing for the first time.

Some time after starting therapy, my face began to show major signs of improvement. My pain had been given a voice. It had been buried and locked very deep within me, but now was encouraged to speak in safe group settings that nurtured and supported my entire body chemistry. It was a slow process. I would improve, then have a little setback and break out in more boils, then improve a little more. As the process gradually picked up momentum, my facial skin began to lighten in color and texture.

I healed physically in one year after that first workshop. There was more for me to learn, however. During the next year the disease tried to reappear, but not on my face. When I went out in public, I would react inside the way I did when the disease was visible. The stress was overwhelming. I felt like I was ready to get on with my life, but my body stayed in reaction for well over a year. I had to relearn how to act with a normal face.

I began to witness the reality of my previous years of trauma naturally undoing itself from the inside out. I experienced what felt like "bizarre" feelings, sensations, and symptoms as my body told its own story of how deeply it had been hurt having held in such enormous inner emotional pain. **It took much longer to heal the body memories of the trauma than it did to heal the disease itself.**

If I had not had the insight and wisdom from having my face healed, I probably would have thought my body's symptoms were new illnesses. I could have even felt jinxed. I felt fearful at times; life wasn't always easy as I hung on tightly to my belief that nature knew how to heal its own, and I was nature's student.

A New Life Revealed

Releasing My Body Memories

God is good! My body memories surfaced at the rate my life was ready for them to be healed. If they had all surfaced at the same time, I would have been overwhelmed. Every body system would have been activated at once to assist my body to eliminate toxins and emotional pain, causing what is known as a "healing crisis." Often people are hospitalized or drugged when this happens, or perhaps, I could imagine, even commit suicide when what is needed most is a welcomed listener to hear the emotional pain.

Body memories appeared as a variety of symptoms, usually when I was about to take on a project or go to some event that was more stressful than was good for me. Welts larger than quarters appeared across my buttocks and sometimes ran down the backs of my legs. White pimples appeared on my lips when I felt pressured. My top or bottom lip would swell up to three times larger than normal. I had flashbacks of traumatic events and cried uncontrollably as my mind replayed them over and over as if they were my current reality.

My lungs hurt. The pressure on my chest was so painful I could hardly breathe; tests showed nothing wrong. Other times I would cough very deeply as if the tight vice grip I had been living in was now releasing. Sleepless nights made me feel like a 90-year-old whose spirit had been sucked out; I was dry inside, hurting, and frail.

Stiff joints and various aches, pains, and low energy continued for a long time; I wondered if it would ever end.

Internalized anger, fear, and rage came out in the form of tooth decay, gum problems, and grinding my teeth. Lack of oxygen in my system from such high, intense stress and deep emotional pain contributed to these problems. Once I began to nurture myself, have a calmer lifestyle, and release my inner pain, these problems improved noticeably.

I had zero tolerance for stress and negativity. I experienced this more when I was in the car, running errands or going to an appointment. I would disassociate and end up on the wrong freeway not knowing how I got there. I would make a list of where I was going and drive right by the location.

I realized the best medicine for me was to rest for as long as necessary. My priorities were to nurture myself and discover who I was spiritually. I had the faith that I would be provided for and I was. I worked only part-time for a number of years, and I was happy that money was no longer my motivator.

I was internally fatigued, but life required certain daily and weekly personal and household chores to be done. On the outside I felt like I looked pretty normal, so I was embarrassed because I felt so weak inside. I could never refuse to do something or just neglect doing it.

I then went through a divorce, which I believe aided my body memories to surface in the aftermath of grieving the loss of my fifteen-year marriage. Divorce was painful, because I went through a natural healing process instead of stuffing the pain. Looking back, though, I can see that the divorce was the vehicle that hastened my recovery time.

My nervous system was short-circuited, and delicate care was necessary to continue to rebuild my energy bank and body. When I violated or depleted my energy, I had no backup reserves. Unfortunately, I had no awareness of when I overextended myself; I suffered from the results often but could not see how I did it. With each overextension I had a setback, sometimes getting very sick and having to start from scratch. Retraining my ambitious racehorse behavior took patience.

I discovered I had exhausted my adrenal system through mental and physical stress. The adrenal glands produce hormones that regulate the blood sugar level in the body, which provides energy for the muscles and brain. With this exhaustion, I could no longer respond to life's normal pressures.

When I would give a talk, I would write out what I was going to say, rehearse for a week or two, and then give my speech—no more, no less. I was not spontaneous, nor could I rely on my wisdom just to trust my thinking to share with people. I never invited people to ask questions; I knew I couldn't sort through my thinking process fast enough to respond intelligently. It took some years to have the confidence to rely on my brain to function properly.

At one point I was so paranoid about my writing or spelling that I claimed to know nothing about either and refused to even try. I usually got others to do it. Through therapy it was suggested I take a college spelling exam to see where I fit. I knew I'd fail, but I took the test anyway. When the results came back, I was amazed to learn that I had passed! This led me to wonder what other erroneous beliefs I had about myself.

One of the very last obvious symptoms lasted for months: an internal, uncomfortable, mysterious trembling that appeared separate from my outer body. Similar to a mild electrical shock, when it ended it felt like "fear" and trauma had been gently shaken out of my cells. The healing results were significant and noticeable, including greater vitality. These symptoms rarely happen anymore.

What I observed about this internal quivering is perhaps the reason many people are diagnosed with diseases that result in trembling, shaking, and/or mild to extreme pain. Could it possibly be our stuffed fears, stress, and inner emotional unhappiness cellularly telling their own story and choosing to break out of bondage? I'm a perfect example of "all that emotional stuff wanting to get out."

This is one of the reasons I encourage myself and others to play by dancing to rock and roll music as a way to assist, release, and loosen our bodies structurally. I wrote a song for the students of a movement class I held called "I'm Going to Dance in My Own Special Way." Maybe I should have titled it "Dance Your Way to Freedom." (See chapter on "Heal by Expressing and Connecting.")

Not everyone agrees with my thinking. Once a retired professional dance therapist who heard my story cautioned me to not dance without having a degreed therapist with me because, in her words, "Your body memories will surface. You'll get emotionally out of control." That was her belief system, not mine. I believe the majority of us know our limitations.

As the experience of the body memories intensified, my body provided me with a way to work through them. I would lie in bed, allowing my body to rock gently back and forth. I felt as though my body was "unwinding." I remembered being in group therapy and rocking my body back and forth for what felt like hours. Some years later my body tended to want to rock sideways. My body was assisting in my healing!

There is a natural life force and intelligence operating at all times in the universe and in our bodies. I saw demonstrated in my own body an inherent natural tendency towards healing, but if I hadn't had the opportunity because of my beliefs to release my emotions, my body would have remained in a state of perpetual stress, and no doubt deformed. After living with prolonged stress and trauma, even my eyes, the windows of my soul, had shut down.

During this reawakening I asked, "What had happened to my feeling safe, secure, and fulfilled?" Where had that part of my sacred spirit gone? What happened to my vast sensory system and nervous system, that part of me that evaluates what I'm feeling, sending messages to and receiving messages from the brain, keeping me healthy and fulfilled? Under prolonged trauma, the messages to my brain had become too overwhelming for the brain to handle. The unresolved trauma then got stored in my body. I was unconscious of this happening, knowing only that my body just "didn't feel right" and had taken on some strange symptoms in the process of healing.

My body would, however, if left to itself, regain its health as a natural process with lots of self-love and nurturing. It would take time, patience, and confidence, remembering that I did not get my body out of harmony overnight. Eventually my body gave me signals of what was needed that assisted me to reunite with myself.

I'm now more curious than fearful about what my body is trying to convey to me. I know anything can improve with enough love, joy, playfulness, and nurturing. This is an opportunity to be compassionate, determined, and self-guided to get beyond physical and emotional pain and to forgive, grieve, heal, and eventually celebrate the spirit set free.

I now feel very differently about who I am as a person. Now if someone asks me, "Who are you?" I want to respond, "I am who I am," letting my joy and inner, gentle spirit radiate outward to be my explanation. Rather than having my titles, accomplishments, and resume be my identity, or trying to convince somebody about who I am with words, I have realized, to my delight, that I am even more than who I thought I am.

I've come a long way and continue to heal my life. The dramatic part of the unwinding process is over, and I've regained more of my inherent natural self. I say "more of," because I have not totally arrived to what I believe is possible in healing my emotional or body memories. My mind is very clear and sharp. I feel like I'm in a brand-new body; I know my face looks like it.

My body is now my teacher. If I experience pain I stop and listen before it has to shout or cause me illness to get my attention. A simple headache might be telling me I have overextended myself. I trust my intuition to do more of what I enjoy and less of what I don't. I now listen to, respect, understand, and nurture the instrument I walk around in. It's been a journey, but I feel more alive and free to be myself.

My body has become my respected friend by allowing my "emotions to be in motion," to be expressed because I'm in tune and listening, rather than ignored and turned destructively inward. My body set me free to be my true natural self.

Some of the therapies I used in moderation included: massage, Reiki, cranial-sacral therapy, visualization, colonics, acupuncture, acupressure, vitamins, juicing, fasting, aromatherapy, seaweed and sea salt, herbal, mud and clay body wraps, and natural hot springs mineral water baths. If the therapy felt good physically and emotionally, I proceeded. If it caused me to feel bad, get sick or lessen my energy, I slowed my pace. Some people told me that in order to heal I had to get sick to get better. I had been sick too long already, so anything I tried I did in small amounts with caution knowing "more" of anything might not be "better." My body responds more positively to healing when I treat it gently.

Summary

Gradually my emotions began to ooze out, but at their own pace. My memories of the trauma came up for healing when it was time. There were never more than I could handle at any one time. My spirit was moving slowly back to the perfection that had always been there. It was an unraveling, unwinding experience, gently getting my life back to wholeness. I continued to give myself permission when necessary to reach out and get support from friends or emotional or physical therapies. The emotional trauma I experienced has taken years to heal.

A decade later I have no scars on my face, and my eyesight has returned to normal. I **knew** that once I was healed, this disease would never recur. Even though my faithful doctors warned me I was only in remission, I was now strong enough to **know** I was set free from my past. I was one hundred percent convinced that once my nervous system and body chemistry got in harmony, I would be healed forever.

It may appear that I'm against the medical profession. If was I wouldn't have contacted so many doctors for their expertise. If I were in an auto accident, I would not hesitate to call a physician. Unfortunately, most of the doctors I contacted were at a loss to understand my problem or propose a solution. At the time there was not much research done on the immune system as there is today. Even as of this writing, doctors still consider rosacea to be incurable.

Thankfully, more medical universities and doctors are opening up to alternative medicine and using a more holistic approach to healing. Many magazines are printing articles about their discoveries. Home remedies using God's natural ingredients that have worked for centuries now are being reevaluated and reconsidered. My dream is that more of us will take advantage of natural healing remedies, treating them with respect and preserving and sharing the gifts of nature, and that each of us will reclaim and take charge of our health.

Dr. Lee's recommendation to find peace within is still my best advice and remedy. All the choices I make now reflect my making this a priority, and it has made the greatest difference in my well-being. Health is the richest possession we have. Wealth, career, possessions, relationships, or learning are too dearly purchased or indulged in if the cost is our vigor, health, happiness, and spirit.

CHAPTER FOUR

Healing Takes Whatever It Takes: Writing My History

Ten years after healing the rosacea, other areas of my life became available to heal in God's perfect, healthy timing. I was convinced I could still experience more joy. Something wasn't quite right. My body felt heavy, as if I was pushing an unknown cloud. My energy level was low; I needed and wanted a breakthrough. Ever willing, I asked myself, "What is next?" I decided to write, to put my life on paper to view it more visually, and then make decisions.

When you read this chapter and contemplate writing your own history, you may feel overwhelmed emotionally, or feel as though you "don't have time." I invite you to write your history in small increments at a time so you won't feel overwhelmed, but rather empowered and enlightened. Later in the book, I provide suggestions on how to get started. Taking a look at our memories is a way to discover the deep-seated, even generational, behavioral patterns and beliefs to which we have bound ourselves. Once you awaken to them, you can also invite positive change and free your authentic spiritual self. For me, the opportunity was too important to miss.

As I began to write, I considered these questions: What had I believed up until now? Do I still want to have these beliefs? Who do I want to be? How different would I act and think if my life worked really, really well? I remember my corporate days, being confident and proud of my leadership. Now, years later, I was ready to reclaim the self-confidence I had lost.

In writing my history I took the necessary time to write every memory and event in chronological order. The process was like pulling a thread on a piece of tapestry. My life slowly started revealing itself. I tried for the most part to be nonjudgmental of others and myself. My memories became available at the rate I was emotionally and physically ready to heal them, and at a time when supportive friends and therapies surrounded me. I was also able to spend a great deal of time in nature as the process unfolded.

As the difficult parts came up, I sorted out the pieces of my history by telling my story over and over and letting the feelings flow. Interestingly, each time I told it more detail was revealed. At times I grieved deeply. What had happened to my inherent spiritual nature—my free-spirited, fulfilled, playful, creative self? Like a connect-the-dot drawing, my past became clearer. Following are the parts of my history that were the most significant and revealing:

Most of my life I never showed any signs of anger unless pushed to the very limit of my tolerance. I avoided angry people at all cost and prided myself on not crying or getting visibly emotional. I had a saying that "if I cried once every ten years, it was once too often." I was always in control and could endure tremendous pressure and stress. Somewhere I accepted the belief that it wasn't safe to go outside the dotted lines and be spontaneous, flamboyant, and outrageous; to have fun, cry, wail, get angry, and laugh. That is what children know so very well. What happened to me?

Where did I learn my structured behavior? My life's training taught me to separate from my feelings. What was it going to take to break through my armor and find the gems that were my birthright: my divine self, waiting for me to discover it? The healing I had undertaken to date had taken layers off my armor, allowing me to be more real. Now I was listing every memory like a detective solving my own mystery.

Up until the time I began therapy and writing my history, I considered my childhood to be fairly normal, consisting of good times and tragedies, just like everyone else's. Childhood happened many years ago, and I thought I had moved on.

However, I had come to understand that our emotional bodies are a direct consequence of our past and how we process fear, trauma, and grief. Unreleased, the feelings tell their story in the physical body through addictions or illness. Having pain brings us back to life; it often takes suffering in the body for us to seek help and health.

As I wrote I saw that I was an extra-sensitive child, gifted with an acute awareness of my environment. I grew up in the country, enjoying a forest as my playground, experiencing seasons of the year, and having animals and their behavior as my teachers.

I witnessed the healing gifts of nature and home remedies made of herbs and natural ointments, thanks to Dr. Maule, my naturopathic, herbalist, holistic family doctor. His home had a sweet smell from all the flowers and plants that hung to dry as part of his holistic pharmacy. This man seemed to never age. Everyone in my family and community relied on him regardless of the ailment. He had special potions to remedy tumors, infections, arthritis, common colds and flu, anything and everything. Dr. Maule responded to others with prayer, singing, and solutions that came directly from nature. This wonderful soul died some 30 years ago, no one in the community could take his place.

When I was about twelve years old, my mother had gallstones. Dr. Maule mixed one of his concoctions, and Mother drank it over several hours. He sat by her bedside, singing and sharing stories. About ten hours later she passed the gallstones, and I got to see them. Within hours Mother was back to her normal routine. During this same period of time a neighbor lady had gallstones and went to the hospital to have them removed. She took months to recover. I just noticed.

Over time I developed a trust and an intuitive sense of knowing, without the ability to express those feelings and thoughts verbally. My spiritual antennas perceived others' feelings without the exchange of words. I was gifted with the ability to see and feel through an extra-sensitive perception. However, unacknowledged and undeveloped, this gift remained dormant until many years later, when I was able to welcome it once more.

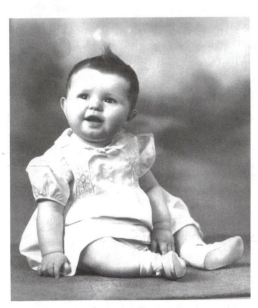

As the firstborn, I was the center of attention and a source of great excitement for the family. I remember my parents and grandparents rocking, singing and playing with me.

My Scandinavian parents had a dream: they wanted four children, a large family like their friends and neighbors. Somewhere between age two and three, my mother started sewing all types of soft-flannel baby clothes and embroidering them with colorful flowers. Mother told me I was going to have a baby sister or brother to play with. Even though I was very young, I knew something wonderful was going to happen in our lives; my mother's sisters all had babies, and now we were going to have our own.

My mother got pregnant three times between my young innocent years of three and six. She had all three babies full-term, two of whom were delivered in the local Catholic hospital, and one in our home by a midwife. Unfortunately all three, two boys and a girl, were either still-born or died shortly after birth.

What happened to my promise of having playmates? My great expectations of having brothers and a sister were abruptly ended. My parents' excitement about having a large family sadly dissipated. Not only did they bury their precious babies, but we also buried our grief, memories, and trauma.

My mother took their death extremely hard for years. Often she mentioned not feeling well, and I felt her grief and mental anguish. A few times a year when her pain would get too great, the two of us would drive into the city, to the chapel in the hospital. Mother would visit with the nuns who had cared for her when she was delivering the babies. I remember the nuns praying with the two of us.

The stained-glass windows of the chapel were very pretty, and the peacefulness and serenity felt very different than anything I had experienced. I liked the nuns. They would tell me stories about the baby Jesus and show me pictures of Him. I could tell they believed that He was a real person, yet I wondered why they never introduced us to Him. They tried to reassure Mother and I that my siblings were with Jesus.

I listened to the nuns and never said a word, but this man Jesus...whoever He was, he made me angry. I couldn't sort out their reasoning; it felt unfair that our babies were with Him and not with our family. Their conversations always left me feeling empty and confused. Because the nuns were older than I was, I didn't think they were lying, but their story didn't make sense and appeared to hurt more than help.

Life after my siblings' deaths was never the same. Our family became very broken and wounded. We lived with extreme sadness and rigidly held the grief inside. Therapy or emotional support was not available. Neighbors and friends had nothing to suggest or offer and moved away from us to avoid their own pain. We became very isolated, never getting to grieve openly, cry, or share our sadness.

Being paralyzed from the shock left only one way to cope with life, and that was to shut the door to the past tightly and stuff the pain. After a while we became so disconnected from our bodies and emotions that there was no awareness of emotional pain.

While there are times when dissociation is valuable and lifesaving, we were chronically cut off from our physical, spiritual, and emotional selves. We each forced ourselves to put on a false face and act differently on the outside than on the inside, separating our emotionally wounded spirits from the world around us. We were unaware of being unaware, and without much-needed support, simply were doing the best we knew how.

Each one of us carried our emotional pain differently over the years. By the time I was in the fourth grade, I had what was diagnosed as rheumatic fever. I believe it was my body's way of burning off the enormous burden I had been carrying, allowing me to be in my body differently from before and giving me some freedom.

The fun-loving child did surface from time to time starting at age eight. After a few piano lessons, I was able to teach myself how to play. I wrote songs, sang, and played for hours with great creativity. Usually I did this when my parents were not at home when I could be a different character, my secret, bright shadow self whom I eventually would allow to emerge.

This expression of emotions and using my voice to sing was very healing. For years I was my own friendly comedian, the opposite of the quiet, reserved, silent child most people saw. Unfortunately, my voice teacher died when I was 16; my cheerleader let me down. That was when I took up my work addiction and never looked back. My natural, musical child died along with my voice teacher. My music stopped.

It was difficult as a young person to accept the death of my young siblings. Growing up in the country, I did not have other children around me for miles to play with. It has taken years of healing for me to embrace my family and inner child—my "core" playful, uninhibited self—with great compassion.

All along my route to healing I tried to figure out what had driven me so hard as a workaholic, almost to self-destruction. By now I had learned that behind every addiction was a cry for help about unresolved issues. Dot by dot, the picture revealed itself.

Disconnected From God

I uncovered a deep core belief that had run my life. I found that losing my siblings set up a huge emotional block to having a belief in a loving God. Could a God who is loving allow innocent babies to die so young? I had to admit that as a young, innocent child I determined that God "had it in" for my family for some unspoken, unexplainable reason. My reasoning continued that if God didn't show us love or favor us by giving me siblings to play with, then my parents and I were somehow less as human beings. I had nowhere to go in my mind but to be critical toward God for my family's supposed punishment.

I didn't have a clue where or who God was, but I was bright enough to understand God was the creator of all things. I felt angry with God for our family's being segregated and treated with such deep disrespect. Being hurt by man was one thing, but to be singled out by the Creator was an insult too great to bear! Hadn't God cut us off, separating us from the joys of a larger family? How else could a child comprehend the enormous shock of losses?

I carried this belief deep within my soul on a subconscious level. My anger felt justified, and no amount of reasoning to the contrary was helpful. I carried years of great embarrassment, hidden shame, and confusion about my relationship with God. I had been incapable of identifying, sorting out, and healing these core beliefs until I began to see them visually on my written pages.

I felt disconnected in church or even out of church. I reasoned that God was out there in the heavens and had so many people to care for that any personal attention to my need was too much to ask.

As I continued to write, I understood why I had been attracted to and married a minister. I wanted so much to feel like a "good person" and do "all the right things." Being a minister's wife was rewarding and one of the hardest assignments I had. I wouldn't consider it an internal "holy" experience. I was still seeking and trying to get the approval of God, and perhaps others in general, rather than establishing a relationship on a deeper, soul level with the Creator.

As the wife of a minister, I noticed how demanding I was in trying to convince others that our religion was the true way to discovering God and judging others' journeys unjustly, as if God didn't know what He was doing. I was gentle, persuasive, and fanatical. I worked hard at being a religious person, following all the rules, and trying so hard to please God and others by being of service. Many times I continued my good works even though I was physically exhausted because "they needed me," rather than being rested and giving for the sheer love of wanting to do something for another. I wasn't balanced enough spiritually to discern when to say yes and no. My addiction to work and my "to do" list didn't stop just because I was in the ministry.

No matter how hard I worked or what I accomplished, my self-critic reminded me I was never ever good enough, or I could have done better. Many times I did work I didn't enjoy but felt I had no choice in the matter. I won top awards and bonuses to prove my worthiness. Only on rare occasions did the critic inside my head allow me to feel loved and supported. My unresolved belief that God had condemned me for the loss of my siblings colored all of my thoughts and behaviors.

I treated myself exactly as I felt my childhood God had treated my family: with rejection. I was overwhelmed by success and oversensitive and crushed by sorrow or criticism—what a combination, of being intelligent and having low self-esteem! When others had urgent business projects, I responded out of my need for approval. However, I never personally acknowledged my abilities so that I could "correct" my self-critic. I was not consciously aware of doing this at the time, but writing my history revealed these innermost patterns and beliefs.

Yet there was a purpose to all this that is beyond my understanding. There was and is a divine timing. The church that seemed to blame my illness on a lack of faith was the same one that led me to the conference where I met Dr. Lee.

Now that I better understood my personality and beliefs, I could determine what I wanted to keep or discard. Re-evaluation was just that. I wanted to validate myself for the areas where I had performed with such distinction, and I also wanted to feel worthy. I had been creative at solving business and health problems, but had never allowed myself self-acceptance and gratitude. I had a lot of catching up to do to be my own cheerleader. It was time to heal my self-critic.

Loss of Trust

The second core belief I excavated was how my fear of failure overrode any enjoyment of my accomplishments. I was unable to trust any long-term success. Bracing myself against the hurt of failure, I never truly got to enjoy the success when it was there. I was so fragile in my spirit that any loss devitalized me, and it was hard to try again. My trust level had been shattered, so I shielded myself.

Where did I learn to not trust? As a tender, innocent child in my formative years, three times in four years I had great expectations of playmates for nine months then was so disappointed when my dreams did not materialize. No wonder I went through life braced so my heart would never, ever be broken again. There was nothing to compare to the deaths in what they had robbed from me.

Having stored my emotional pain and anger deep within my body, I took on the addictive, workaholic behavior in order to feel something. Energy that was not allowed to transform into creativity and joy for living found a destructive outlet. The result was that my addiction, which I intended as a solution, in reality just added another hurt to the ones already had.

Embracing the Possibilities

However, even in this slow, painful process, I was starting to feel more alive and have more possibilities. I was healing my behavior by embracing my worth, uniqueness, and accomplishments. I was now becoming healthy enough to decide to write my own script for the rest of my life. From this day forward I could choose my lifestyle and insist on it. I began to have a vision for the future, including creating my story in book form, trusting God and the angels to see that it got printed and distributed.

I knew I wanted my "religion" to be the way I lived my life and not so much a church or a set of rules. I would learn to talk to myself with as much joy and love as I showed for others. I was becoming more real. The image I held of God and of myself would eventually heal, and I would feel connected and complete in being Georgie. My "beingness" was a delight that I was learning to love. I did not have to prove anything to myself or anyone else.

I have always known I had a purpose on this planet—a contribution to make. After I'm gone, I would like to think I made a difference. My contribution has become a dedication to playing more and using my energy and life as examples for others to follow. Joy, joy, joy. What brought me joy would keep me happy and healthy. "Becoming as little children" is referred to in the Bible. I was becoming untied from my past, freeing up my spirit to experience joy in many forms.

Reconnecting With God

Because my core issues were with God, I decided this was my priority in reprogramming. For the next three years I scheduled my time and desires carefully. I worked part-time and spent every hour I could in nature, three hours at a time when possible. Identifying with God's vast abundance, beauty, detail, and uniqueness and allowing my body to absorb the truth without words slowly moved me out of denial. My body knew the truth, and gradually my mistaken thoughts and beliefs melted away.

I could no longer be in denial about my connection and oneness with the greatness of creation. Just as a glass of water scooped out of the ocean is still part of the ocean, I too was and am very much a part of God. Every detail including my breath was a free gift, and I was now capable of breathing freely and deeply as the pain of my past was forgiven and let go. I learned that I'm sacred and divine, and have a great new awareness of my goodness and capacity for love. I began to have a heart experience with God that filled me with joy from the inside out.

My beliefs about myself and others have completely changed. The one thing I don't do anymore is to judge others' paths of belief, for fear they will influence or contaminate me. I don't place people in boxes of good and bad. I used to do this in my arrogance of playing a false god. I say "false" because I don't believe God judges as much as God sees all people as equal. My own judgment is the only thing that contaminates me. As I have grown in the strength of knowing who I am, others cannot shake my truth.

I'm more centered and healthier than ever before. I am not threatened by attending a meeting, and I do not monitor others' language with a critical ear. Everyone has his or her own truth and individual lessons as part of his or her path. I acknowledge all people as God's people in their own transition, arriving at their own conclusions as I have, in their own divine timing. I see them in this lifetime or the hereafter as being sacred, precious, and good.

Prayer has now become a big part of my life. I constantly ask that our family memories be forgiven and healed. As a result, I have developed increased compassion for my parents and myself as we journey together. We were unable to see from God's higher perspective why God needed three babies in heaven. Perhaps they had a far greater assignment and needed a strong family to release them for their angelic, divine mission. What if the world were made better because of their willingness not to stay, but to do God's will?

I was learning that all things happen for good, despite appearances, and that if God is anywhere, then He is everywhere equally present, even in allowing children to be transformed from death to newness of life for God's glory. My siblings were the chosen ones.

Each person has a path, and I too was a chosen one, but on a different path than my siblings. My experience with illness opened my heart to identify with all people and have great compassion for their circumstances, rich or poor, sick or healthy. I feel very humble and blessed to have lived through this disease. I also feel authentic in my beliefs; the greatest of educational institutions couldn't provide me with what I have learned.

I learned to be with people with a disease and offer them hope, to see the truth of the condition and have no doubt about the possibility of their healing. Knowing what I know, I can be with them with unconditional love and an absence of fear.

Learning to walk gently through life and listening to the voice of God's divine spirit instructing me, I've grown to become more of the precious child—looking, waiting, and respecting God's directions. "Being" my sacred self is more valuable than trying to convince myself I am worthy of love.

I now realize the tremendous benefit and healing that has taken place from writing my history, and it has transformed my life. Later in this book, I will offer ways to help you write your own history when you are ready and divinely inspired to do so.

CHAPTER FIVE

What Caused Me to Stick to My Truth?

The Old Testament talks about people who were prepared and traveled long distances to do battle. Although I didn't know it at the time, I too was being prepared through much of my life. My battle with disease was won, and I will never forget where I've come from. I'm committed with gratitude to the One who led me through it. The direction I chose for finding health answers would have been much more difficult—in fact almost impossible—without my business background. The following describes how I was being prepared and divinely guided, and what I learned that business and health problems have in common.

From childhood, my experience with a naturopathic doctor showed me how health problems could be solved with natural remedies. Also, as an only child with little to distract me, I spent hours observing nature, listening, feeling, and watching. This experience developed my intuition. In nature my inner spirit learned what peacefulness felt like, and I found a welcoming sense of safety and joy. Knowing that the wind had power to destroy or bless, and I soon learned as a young adult that people also had this same characteristic.

By the age of 25 I had begun to trust my inner truths. I was a vice president of a company for which I hired, trained, and managed employees. I helped the company to expand nationally, creating great financial success. At the same time I was hired as an advisor to the board of directors for a 100-year-old company. God placed me there. I felt very young, much like a child among the pros.

God gave me the ability to find solutions for complex problems, mainly because I was capable of listening and trusting my own inner guidance. I was sensitive to people and their environments. I found that principles of finance, marketing, management, employees, and sales were very similar for any type of business or size.

I had the opportunity to challenge my beliefs in many different arenas through my work. One company hired me to manage 175 women from varied cultural backgrounds who were experiencing many conflicts. Their environment was out of control and very negative. Believing in team building, I taught them how to be proud of their actions rather than hurtful, and to strive to bring out each other's inherent goodness. I taught them that no one hurts another unless he or she had been previously hurt. Hurting someone else is a distorted way of asking or needing to be loved. We just keep passing down our pain. I watched these same women triple production in four months and make commitments to learning a better way to live, not just a better way to work.

Over and over my beliefs proved to be accurate. One Fortune 500 company hired me to train its national managers who were almost entirely ex-military personnel. I trained them how to evaluate, understand, listen to, and motivate their employees.

My work showed me that managers, staff, culture, and race create interesting challenges in eliminating the age-old problem of intolerance that exists between and even within the same ethnic groups. Much energy is wasted in the workplace on problems that more than likely have their roots in the teachings and experiences from childhood. I found that in general, people want to create identities and standards that support our sacred commonalities. We all have red blood regardless of our size, sex, or color of skin. We all have been created by the same source. Healing our lives starts with getting our facts straight and stopping the hurt, judgment, and double standards. Healing internally invites a healthier belief system to represent who we are, whether as a company or as an individual.

The training I implemented sought to take the difficulty out of communicating and to encourage all people to succeed and prosper. Employees were supported in developing creative teams that enjoy work, rather than teams built by force and indifference.

What was the common natural response I noticed in any situation? **I couldn't solve a problem unless I knew what it was.** I didn't have a degree or a packaged, "quick fix" formula for this part of my knowingness. I had only my God-given intuitive self. No two business situations were the same, so I always was kept challenged.

I knew in my heart that most business problems were not unsolvable. Even in borderline bankruptcy, a business could be turned around. Therefore, I taught people how to take pride in themselves and have a creative purpose. A company cannot build success and profit by allowing disharmony, negative energy, confusion, disrespect, and distrust to lead, because the result is always confusion and destruction. Peaceful, happy environments create greater profit margins with less effort, allowing the magic and miracles of life to be everyday events. Changing the message changes the results. The principles don't change, but our use or misuse of them does.

In my physical challenges I learned to rely on my inner wisdom to show me that health and business problems had many of the same solutions. Business problems were never labeled "incurable for life." Why should health problems be? Business success was based on principles to be respected; I discovered health was also. I'm a living example.

I helped businesses utilize God's principles that included creating harmony, orderliness, beauty, respect, integrity, and joy—the same characteristics I observed about nature.

As I used my business experience to look at my disease, I saw that, like any dysfunctional business, my disease represented my dysfunction.

* I was out of harmony; physically and mentally stressed out.
* I lost my self-respect; I had a socially acceptable work addiction.
* I betrayed my spiritual integrity; I lost my joy.
* I lacked the beauty and order of living peacefully; I lived in fear.

Through my journey back to health, I've learned a great deal about being compassionate with others who do not know what they do not know. I believe we all have a responsibility to make a contribution to our environment and the world around us. I want to share the good news: life is meant to be good. May we not settle for less, knowing that God is divinely guiding us.

CHAPTER SIX

The Me I've Grown to Love

Something mighty grand, whom I like to call "God," created me. Knowing that was one thing; convincing my body took much longer. Allowing my body to trust again and feel oneness with God as divine and good took time. I'm growing into this peaceful way of living, and I wouldn't trade it for anything. Transformation into my spiritual true nature is a work in progress.

The me I've grown to love now likes looking into a mirror and noticing my smooth facial skin, with no scars or redness to remind me of my past. My vision has returned to 20/20, and my eyes appear very clear. I even get extra pampering at times and receive facials just to remind my face how much I appreciate its willingness to heal. I am able to see my miracle face with its own radiance and beauty.

The child who was such a creative delight, playful and highly spirited, has returned thirty years later. I play guitar, write music, and love to facilitate others to feel music as they sing. We don't read song sheets that rob us of spontaneity. Instead we are free to fill our spirits with continual musical sounds, creating an atmosphere of healing and increased joy. I'm more spontaneous and playful singing or sharing with groups than ever, free to respond in the moment rather than being rigid and rehearsed as I once was.

I deliberately find ways to play. Dancing is one of the many new loves in my life. I encourage everyone to move to music with a partner or without. Voice lessons is another method through which I can expand my breathing capacity and play with making wonderful new sounds, even making nonsense tones that reveal my soul's inner expression and language.

My emotions are also spontaneous. I cry, get angry, laugh, get scared, and experience many other feelings. I label, claim, respect, own, and release these delicious feelings that are my inheritance in keeping me healthy and happy. Being my flexible self, I still reach out for help when I get stuck or shut down, but I notice my recovery time is much faster than ever before.

I walk often to increase my circulation and elimination, walking barefoot whenever I can. I go to the beach and parks to experience the nurturing available in nature. I sit at the beach and write questions in the sand and answer them, amazed at the insights I get. Getting out in the sunshine to increase my vital energy and to remind myself that life is about "shining," I ride my purple and hot-pink bicycle, canoe, swim, and hike, spending as many hours as possible in the great outdoors, especially when I take vacations.

I lean up against trees and treat them like friends. I notice more and more that I'm connected in the moment, because I'm more rested and have released my spiritual self. Butterflies circle around me and even land on me, and we appear to have a kinship. I have a deep love for all critters and animals.

All God's people are my sisters and brothers, so I include relationships with cross-cultural people of all ages in my life. I share my talents for the joy it gives me and ask to be surrounded with people, places, things, and thoughts that are divinely meant for me. I also ask to have discernment about where my time, energy, and efforts are best utilized.

I now notice something interesting when I am with my friends and family. Some of us share openly with each other, speaking freely from our hearts and sharing our growth, fears, tears, joys, and personal discoveries. I feel more energetic, alive, and expansive with them, and my fears begin to fade. With others I get to share no more than the cover of the book of their history or certain pages in their lives. I notice the surface conversation, and I feel less joy. Maybe some day it will be safe for us to get closer.

For some I'm a prayer partner and for others a cheerleader. I absolutely believe without one doubt that prayer works. I'm on a prayer team as a way of serving and giving to others in gratitude for all of my blessings. Volunteer work helped lead me back to feeling personal value. It is love going around in a circle, giving and receiving. When the opportunity arises, I do guided prayer and meditations with others that are very vivid, using the imagination to remind us of our oneness with God's beauty, love, and perfection. Upon request I do "sacred blessings" with people for their lives and dedication of events such as homes, land, project, relationships, career, etc.

I believe that God, Jesus, Mary, Holy Spirit and angels are alive and real in my everyday life and willing to help me if only I will ask. Until I had positive demonstration, I would never ask because I didn't believe. I know now I'm worthy, and asking and receiving guidance is a way of life.

I was privileged to be the national marketing director and health educator for an international organization that offered eight-week workshops on preventing major health issues. These workshops were taught in hospitals, corporations, universities, and a variety of churches. I also have studied and practiced as a licensed massage therapist and instructor with emphasis on cranial work (working with the head and nervous system). For about twenty years, while traveling across the United States, I've witnessed many people healing what others thought was impossible, and I'm convinced healing can happen.

My Joys In Life

My greatest joy in life is facilitating others who are eager to learn about their bodies and sincerely willing to release dysfunction and embrace wholeness. It is a big commitment and it is not always easy, but the rewards are worth it. I do telephone consulting with some and visit in person with others. I share the possibility of bonding with the wounded child and nurturing her/him to remember that they have their own self-repair healing available, should they choose to reclaim it.

I do more of what I love, always striving to stay in joy. I rest and monitor my energy closely so that I don't give my energy to projects and people out of exhaustion. I want to continually increase my sacred energy bank, and give others only my overflow. Money and all good things flow more freely when I stick to this principle.

The focus of my future is in the healing ministry. I have evolved into a playful person who can laugh, use humor, and also be tender, gentle, wise, feeling equal with anyone and everyone. I'm growing into being a storyteller, using my vast experience to capture others' imaginations to share in the vast possibilities available for all of us in healing, careers, etc. I invite people to share their stories including their hurts, pains, victories, and hearts' desires.

My Family

I'm very fortunate that both my parents are alive and I'm getting to embrace each of their lives. The more I've healed, the more compassion I have for them and the extreme losses they experienced with my siblings' deaths and various other hardships they endured without therapy or support. As I have explored my past, I have not only uncovered traumatic memories, but lovely ones as well. Reconnecting to both have been a great treasure.

From our humble beginning of living in a two-room house with an outdoor toilet, I never considered that I grew up in poverty. We definitely had little money at times, but we lived abundantly off of nature and the earth. We grew vegetables in a garden and had wild game for meat. Mother sewed all my clothes.

I attended a country school, two classrooms for grades one through six, where two teachers taught 70 students all required subjects.

My father started his own business as a heating and plumbing contractor when I was seven and became very successful. He owned one of the largest companies in a small town. My mother was his secretary, bookkeeper, and bill collector.

When I was eight, my parents built a new home on two acres of land. They had trees from their land made into lumber that created a beautiful country home, surrounded with forest and wildlife. My parents are now in their eighties but still live on this wonderful homestead and have a great respect and love for the outdoors.

Mother taught me how to be a fine seamstress. During my younger years I won many local awards, proudly modeling my own designs and clothing. As a family we spent hours together fishing in crystal clear blue waters, enjoying our weekly trophies, small or large. For many years we planted small pine trees on our land amongst the forest as part of a conservation program for young people, and I have gotten to watch them grow.

For junior and senior high, I attended school in the city, where I was surrounded by hundreds of young people. I was introduced to my love for chorus and volleyball and the delight in having my own car.

My family still owns what we call our "sanctuary in nature," twenty-two acres of beautiful lush forest about fifteen miles away from our home. This land holds many fond memories; my mother walked to and from school with her eight siblings through trails that are still there today. My mother and father have hunted deer all of their married life, enjoying this parcel of land. This is where I played in the forest, and where I still enjoy walking. In this environment I embraced my sensitivity to nature, as did my parents and their families, who are still deeply rooted in the area.

I'm a third generation Scandinavian who, two weeks after high school graduation, moved to another state to explore my education and career. My gypsy character had a desire for adventure but also needed room to breathe after living with so many losses.

My parents were exactly the right parents for me. Even though I was their only living child until age seventeen, they allowed me to be who I was and do what I wanted to do. With some hesitation, they gave their blessings as I ventured out of their nest. It must have taken great strength on their part to acknowledge my wishes and to let me go.

My Parents' Compassion and God's Miracle Child

When I was sixteen, my parents volunteered to care for a one-year-old baby boy named Bob. He had received brain damage from abuse that resulted in a fall, had cerebral palsy, was paralyzed from the waist up, and couldn't cry. The doctors said he could possibly die within the week. Through long hours of care and love Bob survived.

My parents' long-time dream of having another child in their lives was coming true, and they adopted him.

God performed many miracles on my new baby brother. Doctors said he would never walk or talk, but at age three he did both. His head was misshapen, and my mother was taught how to take her hands and reshape his soft small head back to normal. Through eye surgery Bob's eyes were stabilized, so he could see without his eyes floating opposite each other and rolling back into his head.

Up until the age of five, because of his brain damage, the doctors said he could die at any moment. He lived! During those years, because of his condition, my parents and I lived on edge twenty-four hours a day. God gifted this frail, sickly child with a natural musical talent that surpassed all his weaknesses. He was a born musician. When Bob was six, my parents bought him his first organ. By age nine he was playing in churches, and at age fourteen he won a music scholarship. Eventually he made a career as a church organist and choir director.

He died at age 42. Throughout his life he was in and out of intensive care and not expected to live until morning, but he did—one miracle after another. Before his death he swung on death's door for five years with a terminal disease, yet always maintained a great sense of humor about his ability to continually survive. God held Bob's hand as the rest of us watched him walk on the fine edge of life and death.

Because of my own healing, I had a strong desire to see my brother healed. He didn't heal physically, but actual death was his healing, leaving him free to be with angelic musicians. He allowed my family and me to grieve his dying process over a long, time, preparing us for his transition.

My brother and I were so close that when he first was placed in intensive care and not expected to live, the thought of losing him revived the pain I felt when my three other siblings died. I didn't want to feel the pain, but it erupted in other ways. Once I even disassociated for two months, living numbed out and going through the motions of life while internally hysterical. When I finally got my life back together, I felt as though I had been in a time warp. Everything around me was piled up from being neglected. I didn't think I would ever be strong enough to experience his death. When he did die, I was finally able to embrace his life and even sing at his funeral, sharing his wonderful life's story. Time heals.

At his death my parents and I were able to grieve the years of losses we had never been capable of grieving until now. We wept together, healing our deep hidden hurts and starting life all over. My brother will always be part of our lives and spirits.

Marriage

Wanting to be part of a family, I had been married twice with no children when the angels sent me yet another husband, William "Dub" Holbrook. He has four children, eight grandchildren, and even great-grandbabies. That makes me a stepmother and grandmother without ever being pregnant. Being invited into someone else's large family circle has helped me learn to continue seeking what is truth for myself while keeping an open mind for others' beliefs and behaviors.

Marriages have helped me redefine my definition of "soulmate:" Two souls mate, making it easier for each other's soul to evolve. Enhancing each other's life allows each to reach his or her full potential. They respect and honor the significant part of the other's divinity on this journey. They never deliberately discount or hurt each other. Seeing the goodness or faults in others only reflects what we think about ourselves. It takes people who are balanced emotionally, spiritually, physically, and mentally to be complementary of each other, enhancing, not destroying, their individuality or relationship.

To experience more of me I've chosen partners who have helped me heal, be challenged and grow in ways I couldn't by myself.

My partners have come from different backgrounds, yet I've learned that the bonding glue that makes a marriage come alive and last is having and enhancing ways to communicate. To be with someone who is willing to feel safe talking about secret thoughts and feelings gives the listener permission to learn something valuable about themselves and open up, accelerating the bonding and personal growth. Facts and feelings aren't twisted and held back as in surface conversation. The first step is to choose someone whom we consider our closest and dearest "friend," building a relationship of integrity, honestly, trust, and closeness, continually creating fun times together. Without this we live as strangers.

Love withers without spiritual roots. Without taking time for spiritual growth, only the fruits of the intellectual, financial, and material world remain, of which there will never seem to be enough.

I wondered for years how marriages that look so materially sound could feel so empty. I now know from cherishing my own spiritual growth that spirituality is the missing connection.

I'm really God's soul mate, ready for even greater transformation and relationships.

Growing Gracefully

My age to me spells wisdom. I've grown to stop all body hatred and disapproval. My inner child is now older and far wiser. I love her and would never deliberately harm her or put her down ever again. I want to be an example of aging, allowing my body to tell and show the story of my life as it unfolds. I no longer need to hide because it seems I'm not beautiful enough to please people. I think about what it would be like to live without mirrors, media, or significant others to impress.

If I close my eyes and ask myself, "How old am I?" I don't really know if I'm twenty-nine or fifty-nine years old. My soul never ages and continues to be youthfully free. I enjoy my female friends as we support each others' healing, and especially the honor of getting older and acknowledging our great feminine wisdom of honoring all people. We have dropped hurtful competition around age, the latest fashions, body shapes, finances, and education, and being subservient in any way to the same or opposite sex. The me I've grown to love feels more beautiful and wise inside as life goes on.

"Great feminine wisdom" describes my friend, soul sister and teacher Linda B. She taught me the God-given natural healing process described in the next chapter, "Collect Your Inheritance." Implementing this process into my life has been inspirational, insightful and healing, and to this very day continues to be one of the greatest gifts in my own recovery.

I want more "Lindas" in my life. These are people who have a calling to make the world a better place, with no turning back or leaving it up to others; who are willing to heal enough layers of their own lives to be supportive of others; and who are good listeners, giving others permission to trust their own healing, inherent desires, thinking, and goodness. I want to know more people like Linda, who treat others like a supportive universal family, touching the hearts of those in the work-place and in their homes, and who acknowledge people as valued and unique, celebrating both our differences and commonalities. I am so grateful for the limitless opportunities and possibilities that await all of us as we join hands together.

The outrageous, flamboyant side of me that was dormant for years keeps awakening and must be expressed to keep me really alive! It is never too late to start doing those things that truly excite me from the inside out. Fairy tales are more and more a part of my reality now. On my third date with Dub, I had an opportunity to feel like a real princess. He bought me a gown, a designer, full-length princess dress. We danced at the Grand Mardi Gras Ball at a very elaborate hotel. The playful dancer emerged from me to create a new life.

I believe I am a spirit in a human body, expressing myself in the moment, spontaneous and free. I am no longer threatened by what others think. My soul calls me to walk my truth. My self-critic speaks up less often, and I address it straight on. It only lasts minutes now and doesn't destroy me. I'm growing into loving myself more.

I stand as an example of healing the seemingly incurable and encourage others wanting to break out of limitations into a spirit set free. I bring my gift of perseverance, faith, and hope to others.

My talents are many. I'm free now to pray, sing prayers, spiritually coach, hold sing-alongs, write music, play my guitar, tell stories, give a sermon, or teach on health. My life has been a journey of being led and guided to greater truth and awakening. I continue to learn as I heal and with health comes a responsibility to live more than talk what I've learned.

Dreaming about My Future

My fantasy about my older years is to locate a beautiful parcel of wooded forest where people can experience being out in nature with trails, ponds, fountains, and flowers. I will have a chapel built on this land where all people and cultures can experience silence and stillness, peace and harmony. An unspoken but powerful love will permeate the chapel and the grounds.

I will live on such a property with my family, with open doors for the community to join us, never shutting off from the world or from seekers and guests. I can see myself joyfully smiling, singing, and sharing the wisdom, books, music, and materials of my years here on earth with others who want to be playmates to do the same. I want to continue living in harmony with nature the way I grew up. My greatest dream is to leave a living memorial, allowing my efforts to be utilized for future generations.

My friend, I have told you who I am and shared my innermost thoughts. I hope you have gained and gleaned some insights for yourself. I would be thrilled if you received one thing from my story that changed your life.

My story doesn't end here. The following chapters include information I found to be helpful in order to heal and stay healthy. Try some of the ideas and experience why and how they became meaningful for me. Some of these ideas will be useful for you now, and others may become part of your life later on. Take what has meaning for you, and leave the rest.

We are being called to remember better how much more we really are.

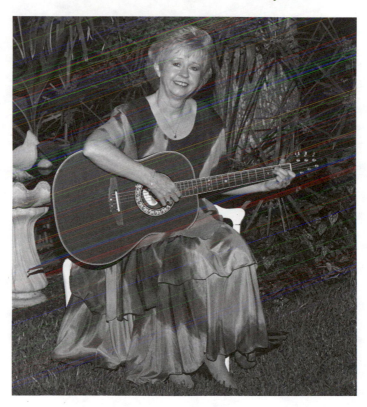

PART II
Your Spiritual Self

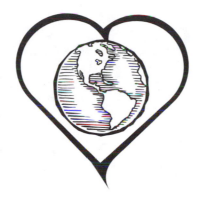

This section of the book includes how to acknowledge, develop, trust, and live spiritually.

By divine intervention I was led to spiritual teachers who showed me that I had a concept of God that led to separation, and who taught me how I could **experience** God.

My life has been one of remembering, forgetting, and awakening.

I hear your voice
I can open my eyes,
breathe deeper,
and feel secure,
knowing I am loved.

May those like me who have been thirsty for a deeper experience learn to apply their own innate wisdom in being part of God's Oneness, never to thirst again.

CHAPTER SEVEN

Collect Your Inheritance
True Story or Fable? You Decide

God, the all-wise Eternal Spirit, created the earth. From center to circumference God is equally present. This same fathomless spirit delights in exquisite precision and detail. Having infinite ideas and resources available, this spirit creates, using love as the ingredient molded into various shapes and forms. Principles as accurate as mathematics are available for us to use as an "owner's manual" for life.

From the beginning of time, universal knowledge and technology were always advancing and expanding, allowing people to use the vast resources from the land and sky. People utilized the accuracy available, predicting twenty years in advance when the sun would come up in any given area, down to the very second. Confusion was not an ingredient in life. Farmers could plant carrots with certainty, knowing carrots would be harvested.

Human bodies, uniquely created as individual masterpieces, received fingerprints unlike anyone else's. Samples of blood, saliva, hair, and skin had unique, symbolic codes. Some even had different blood types than their mothers or fathers. Each person embodied different likes, dislikes, personalities, purpose, cultures, languages, and talents to enhance the richness available in sharing and complementing each other.

With detailed mastery, God installed a direct internal guidance system in each child for direct communications with the Beloved. It is impossible ever to separate or extinguish the soul from its maker; this all-wise spirit wouldn't want it any other way.

First and foremost, your identity was a "divine idea." Your soul, life force, and body were developed out of the intelligence of the infinite. Beginning at conception your parents' thoughts, actions, diet, and environment contributed to the start of your physical, emotional, mental, and behavioral patterns, beliefs, and sense of well-being. In the birthing womb of your mother, you were safe, protected, rocked, and nurtured as God's masterpiece developed.

You were given a highly sophisticated body and brain, sensitive to the actions of the grown-ups around you and stimulated by their touch, smells, tones of voice, and emotions.

Self-Expression Becomes Limitless With Encouragement

In an ideal environment you were welcomed into this world and confirmed as being special. Lullabies were sung to you. Your name was whispered in your ears. You were rocked and pampered, bathed and clothed. You were treated as a precious, priceless treasure. Your family avoided any and all shocks or frightening experiences to your infant, tiny body; every need was taken care of, respecting your every whimper.

As an infant you could do nothing wrong; dirty diapers, spitting up, crying, wailing, and making angry noises were all natural body releases and expressions. Everything you did was welcomed.

Your parents allowed you to be significant, so at two or three years old, you were able to rely on your creative, vivid imagination to build your dreams as you played with imaginary situations, delightfully creating with cardboard boxes, dolls, cars, trains, pots, and pans. It took very little to entertain you or for you to feel contentment and happiness. Every chance you had, you played, adding sound effects to discover the genius within you.

Your mind, if allowed, developed, utilizing its ingenious wisdom so that with a little encouragement, you could have learned several languages. You noticed qualities, characteristics, and important aspects of other cultures to be respected and admired. The opportunity to have dress rehearsals and get to play the part of another child's life opened up greater possibilities of learning and appreciation. Singing and dancing to a variety of music from other cultures inspired you to see people of the world as your brothers and sisters. Older children taught you how to create, play safely, and enjoy games in which everyone could win.

You might have been taught no limits, walls, fears, or hate to stifle the Infinite's masterpiece.

Divine creativity expanded as you trusted the images you saw in your mind as ideas. This was of uppermost value, developing your self-confidence, intuition, and faith in your own abilities. You might even have seen, heard, and talked with angels, having them as celestial friends and helpers.

As a child you stayed in motion and movement. It was not only fun but vital to your every organ and cell, assisting your body by cleansing and moving out waste products, allowing your body to stay healthy. Playfully you kept your body flexible and buoyant; you enjoyed running, rolling, twisting, jumping, dancing, and climbing. You were totally spirit in a human body, and you were, as your natural, outrageous self, a delight to be observed.

In an ideal situation school was very exciting, helping you develop your inherent skills. You were encouraged to listen within yourself and trust your own intuitive likes and dislikes. You were taught what you needed to know in order to function in society. You were never forced to learn against your will or study subjects not suited for you. You chose your own chair and went to the bathroom when your internal urge beckoned you. Every classmate was treated with dignity and respect regardless of race, culture, size, gender, sexual preferences or color of skin. You had teachers who helped to expand everyone's individual preferences and uniqueness.

Your teachers and family were your personal cheerleaders in helping you reach your full potential. They acknowledged the doorway to your personal empowerment and happiness. What brought you joy, love, play, creativity, and fulfillment was important. They encouraged you to share your frustrations, joys, fears, insights, suggestions, achievements, and discoveries, allowing you to experience your natural healing processes. They listened to you use your imagination and express your ideas. They supported you in looking for ways to create in goodness, love, usefulness, and betterment. You were respected for recognizing opportunities to improve and serve, and to give in order to receive. You felt secure and loved because your family and friends could be counted on. You absolutely were taught that work and play are one and the same, as are health and happiness.

In our story, you are now a teenager. The natural healing process has always been welcomed. When you get emotionally stuck or shut down, there is a caring person available who is very sensitive and aware of how to assist you. You are encouraged to talk and release feelings while another gives his or her delighted attention with no interruptions or advice. You talk, sharing your story, explaining in every detail what is bothering you. Your feelings unravel. Your hands are perhaps cold and sweaty. You might have a nervous knot in your stomach. Breathing fast or shallow, you might cry, yawn, or raise your voice in rage as you share. Eventually your hands and body are warmer and the knot is gone, reflecting that emotions have been expressed and released. Centered and stable, your clear thinking is regained; you are once again capable of figuring out your own solutions. You are grateful for having a supportive person who didn't give advice, interrupt you, or have a need to tell you their stories while you were the one in need.

If your support person is clear of his or her own emotional distress or can put it on hold, he or she is able to listen to your every word, remembering details and being fully present rather than reacting from their own unresolved past. Allowed and encouraged to express and release your emotions, keeping them in (e)motion and not stuffed, your attitude about life is connected, confident and self-empowered. Clear thinking and sensory awareness enable you to utilize your vessel knowing that, with your inheritance, "details matter," allowing your inner senses to "know" that you know, absolutely respecting your soul's likes and dislikes.

Results of Denying Our True Natures

Few of us were raised in this ideal situation, however. Most of us learned to begin to violate the natural healing process almost from birth, and definitely by age two.

At that magical age of two and still feeling special, you were exceptionally curious, innocent, inquisitive, and brilliant. Perhaps one day you ventured hurriedly to check something out and tripped on a sharp corner of the end table. Down you went to the floor, knee bruised and hurting. You responded by crying and wailing. Hearing you, a family member picked you up. This big person's thoughts and intentions got conveyed through their voice, which told you what to do to feel better:

* There, there, don't cry.
* Here is a piece of candy; you'll feel better.
* Big boys/girls don't cry.
* It is not that bad. Look! I'll kiss it and make it better.
* Stop crying!

They may have even hit you. You were encouraged not to feel or show your emotions. Therefore, you internalized the hurt. If this only happened once in a lifetime, it would go unnoticed; unfortunately, more often than not this scenario gets repeated often over many years.

If someone had given you his or her undivided attention, looking into your eyes and allowing you to feel his or her sincerity while you cried and wailed, your body would have released the trauma by heating up or trembling. Healing would have occurred more rapidly, perhaps even with little or no bruising. Releasing the sadness, fear and anger from a physical hurt allows healing to take place more rapidly.

Unfortunately the caregivers around you may not have been informed, or may have been too busy to notice or protect you and encourage your natural responses. Like most of us, they trained their "natures to be unnatural;" while needs for food, shelter, and clothing were met, their emotional/spiritual lives and natural healing process were ignored and not valued, embraced, or welcomed.

To you as a child, big people appeared as giants; surely they knew better than you. You were treated as "just a kid" and told to be "seen and not heard," as if you didn't have feelings or even likes and dislikes, instead of being seen as intelligent, special, and worthy of respect. After awhile it became harder to have your own personal respect and identity.

Your mind and body have seen, felt, and recorded all, and are capable of storing years of unexpressed emotional pain and negative body memories of every event, smell, color, taste, sight, and sound. The mind and body are almost like a movie film, storing every detail. After awhile you react to anything or anyone who reminds you of your past. Some people even have memory loss of their early childhood in order to function in spite of hurts and humiliation.

Understanding the Results

The hurt of prejudice, jealousy, selfishness, judgment, and abuse are passed down through each generation. Eventually people, societies, and standards are lowered; the social system gets broken down, and people have no respect for each other. It becomes more difficult for people to function or override their emotional pain and distresses. Eventually they find it hard to care or be of service, giving up and numbing out. None of God's children would intentionally hurt another if he or she hadn't learned that behavior from being mistreated themselves—if he or she had not learned from their early formative years about feelings of self-doubt, unworthiness, and self-abusive behavior. We would have healed if we had been listened to well.

You become molded into the patterns, beliefs, and behavior of those around you, for better or worse. You find it difficult to know who you are, what you want, or how to win, appear to have no purpose or to have lost it, or you became competitive, aggressive and numb, driven by addictions. Your body then shuts down as a natural response to protect your incredible guidance system. It cannot respond and function when your "inherent true nature" has been denied or betrayed long enough.

Once shut down, perhaps starting at a young age, you may take on an addiction of work, food, drugs, sex, alcohol, excessive spending, excessive drive for education, or anything that alters your feelings or allows you to escape feelings and numb the pain. You stay in situations that increase your stress, lower your vitality, and zap your very life force because you have a core belief that "it's impossible to change" or, "I feel I'm not OK and I will continue to prove it" or, "money or my addictions are more important or valued than my health and happiness."

You pile the addiction on top of an already emotionally shut-down body. No amounts of activity, possessions, or addictions bring you peace of mind. Eventually your body appears to turn against itself, rebelling with pain, illness, disease, loss of memory, low energy, weight gain or loss, and discouragement. Society has locked you in; there is no logical way to get out, to go home. Relationships, career and financial losses or successes all pull you in many painful directions.

Through tragedy, turmoil, disappointments, and failure, your life "hits bottom." You choose not to suffer one moment longer; you give up! You might even have to fight for your life from what feels like your deathbed. You are tired, so very tired of having a wilderness experience and not going anywhere special. With no one to direct your dissatisfaction, you don't understand what is lacking, but you feel very empty and separated from God and life.

Your body and health have been trying to get your attention, whispering to you: "There is a better way." Your life gets interrupted, and you are forced to stop! Your body longs to remember how pleasant, secure, safe, and totally fulfilled you would like your life to be.

There are many roads and paths that lead you back home in your heart. God has beckoned you. Your inheritance is waiting, sad that it took you so long. Soon you will never, ever need or want an addiction or destroying behavior to cover up your pain or hurt. You start learning and doing whatever it takes to reclaim your sacred self in all its fullness.

Your Inheritance: The Natural Healing Process

You will always be the divine idea of God with Spirit at your core, striving to direct you. Listening for directions gets easier or harder depending on your life's training. But we can relearn.

The masterpiece of your body, your sacred vessel, is worthy of acknowledgment, specially designed to stay in superb harmony allowing the inlet and outlet of the spirit's divinity, love, and breath to flow. The Maker has equipped you to keep you basically healthy and maintenance free, with precision and balance. Minute details were considered in creating you such as your body temperature, which for most of us remains constant at 98.6 degrees even in the hottest or coldest of conditions. Deviations would indicate attention was needed to your health.

You are an individual masterpiece, yet with similarities to acknowledge "oneness with all people having the same spiritual source." All people unless physically damaged are born with the same inheritance of having a natural healing process available; its response is written in the memory of every body cell and fiber, evaluating, identifying, feeling, releasing, and always allowing the body to process the emotions and come back to "center." All of this is automatic, although we are often unaware of it.

It is natural for our bodies to respond spontaneously to sensory stimuli, joys, and fears. This response activates as one experiences pain, hurt, illness, shame, embarrassment, personal violation, humiliation, physical or sexual abuse, stress, fear, loss, success, achievement, excitement, joy, praise, great anticipation, recognition, celebration, etc.

Inherent in the body is an internal "natural healing process" that allows us to release our emotional feelings as we encounter everyday experiences, so we can stay healthy and emotionally balanced.

* It is a natural physiological bodily response.
* It is the language of emotions that gets felt and released.
* It is the way we experience great feelings and release unpleasant ones.

Following are two examples of everyday encounters and potential emotional responses:

1. I attend a party and only know the host. I arrive and feel very out of place. A complete stranger initiates a conversation, asking a tactless, personal question about my friend who's hosting the party. I feel intimidated. I start talking nervously, my hands start to sweat, and I feel uneasy and tense as I respond. Then I notice my body feels chilled and I'm physically very uncomfortable. The conversation ends and within a short period of time these symptoms go away.

If we take a closer look at what just happened, we can better understand the spontaneous, natural way to release feelings:

* Rapid talking releases my embarrassment and anger.

* My body chills and cools down, releasing my fear.
* My hands sweat, indicating I'm feeling anger. Sweating also releases the anger.
* I feel better; I have let my body respond.

2. Someone who I care about a great deal disappoints me. I want to cry, but choke down the tears, pretending I didn't notice. My mind races, rehearsing my disappointments. Within a short period of time, I have a knot like feeling in my stomach and blame it on the food I ate.

   In this instance, the natural healing response is denied:

* My first feeling is to want to cry, demonstrating my sadness about the situation.
* I stop the natural response of crying, I swallow and deny my feelings.
* My "stuffed emotions" get internalized, violating the natural healing process.
* I feel horrible. Over time, the stuffed emotions may reappear in the form of physical symptoms.

Everyday incidents arouse natural feelings and emotions	Feelings and emotions spontaneously will release themselves
Grief or tears of joy	Crying
Embarrassment	Laughter
Embarrassment, light fear, anger	Rapid talking and laughing
Fear	Trembling, urinating more than usual
Releasing anger	Loud talking
Anger	Sweating
Body heats up for anger	Body heat facilitates the emotional release
Body feels cold when holding in fear	Body trembles to facilitate the emotional release
Releases physical tension held in body	Stretching, scratching, twitching or yawning

Feelings are to be felt and released. In infinite perfection the healing process, when honored, allows the body to return to balance and harmony. If the healing process is violated, ignored, denied, or not utilized, the emotions get "stuffed." The body system reflects the results by becoming devitalized in some way.

The body's level of balance is reflected in the human aura. The dictionary describes the aura as an invisible emanation or energy field that surrounds all living things. This state can even be seen and photographed with special cameras as the human aura glows about the body, beautifully radiating colors, reflecting the essential well-being of the interior. Auras vividly reveal our spiritual, physical and mental well-being. Pictures of holy people have been portrayed with luminous halos or auras.

In a state of well-being, the aura expands and brightens. In a state of internal discomfort, dissatisfaction, violations, or hurts, the aura will shrink and even discolor. Eventually with enough emotional dis-ease, the physical body will become ill.

Collect Your Inheritance

You deserve to collect and reclaim as much success, happiness, health, playfulness, joy, and love as you can imagine. They are your birthright. Start expressing your feelings, choosing wisely what will bring you joy. Trust your own inherent intuition, learn the natural emotional healing process, and start observing your internal body language by honoring and respecting your sacred body.

Soon you will start seeing the gift of your longings, dissatisfactions, emptiness, and pain; they were trying to get your attention to redirect you "as if turning you towards the sun." Thank goodness the damage didn't go too far.

Each individual masterpiece is special to God, and your own inner guidance is the one true source to be respected with great integrity and honesty. Your intuition can be one hundred percent accurate once you learn to get in tune with the eternal, wise spirit who created you. Build your confidence in a kinship that wants the very best for you always. Every good thing shall be added unto you. You will be rewarded for being true to your own feelings and seeking freedom, passion for your purpose, and talents following your heart.

Your inheritance is waiting. Like a ripple effect in the water, as you collect and make a difference in your world, you will give others permission to seek their own full inheritance. Admire and cheer them on as your brothers and sisters, being equal with all others, blending cultures and people together as one giant, magnificent tapestry, the real masterpiece created by the Master. Its value is in being whole. It was never intended to be torn into bits and pieces, distorting the picture and dividing against itself, but rather it is intended to show respect for God's wisdom and creation.

Becoming Older and Wiser

The tremendous advantage we have of recognizing our natural dignity and spirituality is at our peak experience, the grand finale of our life. In our advanced years we have the opportunity to become acquainted with our deeper selves that lie beyond the distractions of everyday life.

The possibilities of the mystical and miracles are hinted at in many life experiences that get too little attention because of our busy pace, pushing the river of life opposite its natural flow. Hopefully we can learn to walk through life peacefully within rather than always stressfully, controlling and forcing life to conform to our distortions.

How Do We Want to Spend our Last Days on Earth?

Those who have lived collecting their inheritance, using and acknowledging the natural healing process, are the ones who have been allowed to be emotionally expressive along the way. Those who have learned to savor and experience solitude, enjoying silence and stillness, reassure themselves daily and weekly that they "walk not alone" through life. Instead they cherish living with the familiarity of divine guidance. Many times they have peak experiences of having a deep knowing about things. Having lived their lives with happy heart experiences, they need doctors less often, allowing them to increase their faith in death's transformation, being carried in the arms of the Almighty as a butterfly leaving the shell of the dried-up cocoon behind.

If, through life's training, a caterpillar were the classroom study (as compared to human life), we would observe it building a cocoon by following its inherent instincts. With anticipation we would wait for the birth of a beautiful butterfly. How much fear of the unknown would you have? Has the caterpillar died or been transformed? The butterfly says goodbye to its caterpillar friends to be welcomed into "heavenly bliss" with the freedom to "fly," demonstrating the ingenious mind, precision, and timely life-and-death creation of the Eternal One.

Be a Proud Recipient of Your Inheritance

Whatever your age, it is never too late to change. Start by noticing where you are and where you would like to be. Write your own owner's manual. Decide what you want to believe and what you want your life to represent. Include spirituality, emotional healing, building healthy families and relationships, God, death, improving the environment, stopping oppression, etc. Include the type of mentor or help you may want to enable you to discover more about your beliefs and patterns, helping you to re-evaluate and identify more of the "true you." Pick the subject and write with your new awareness about how you will strive to invite healthy, positive changes in your life.

Upon your death your money will be spent. The only long-lasting, real wealth you can leave behind is your character and the relationships you have touched, directly or indirectly, contributing to future generations as the marriage ceremony so wonderfully states it: "for better or worse."

God has all the time in the world for you to "claim your inheritance" and learn about your life as a divine masterpiece. Welcome the gift.

PART III
Holistic Remedies

Next are experiential holistic remedies that I practice and teach, summarized to gently remove past and present obstacles and open to new, Joy-Full possibilities.

To you, my friend, let us begin.

CHAPTER EIGHT

Daily Practice: "Health" Yourself

When you begin any program that will benefit your body, begin in moderation and gentleness, always being aware of how you are feeling and being careful not to overextend yourself. Too many people want a quick fix and lower their endurance by overexerting themselves. The following are nature's doctors and require little to no expense. You may want to check with your own medical doctor before attempting any of these.

Walking

One of the simplest remedies for almost any ailment is a walking program. Select a suitable distance for yourself and get started, daily if possible. Add to that distance each time you walk. Walking should be enjoyable. Select parks and paths that connect you with nature, and still your mind so you notice your surroundings and their beauty.

Exercise builds and tones the body to strengthen its endurance and keep it fit and in shape. Swing your arms and create a happy walking step. One indication of a good cardiovascular walk is sweating, which releases toxins. This will help your elimination and circulation. Walk alone or with a friend or group. Rest when you need to.

Walking can provide additional benefits. For example, exercise is the last thing we want to consider if we are in pain. However, pain is often the body's way of getting our attention. The greatest relief from pain can come from taking a walk, breathing deeply, and allowing oxygen to be invited in to relieve distress. Exercise can help our minds to get quiet so we can nurture ourselves, reevaluate our situation, and listen to our inner wisdom.

Before I healed layers of emotional trauma, I felt exhausted after just a little exercise. I went through the motions but was unaware that my body was actually emotionally weighed down, so I didn't notice much of a difference.

Now I notice when I walk for three to four days in a row, I feel sharper mentally and accomplish more with less effort. I have greater self-esteem, higher energy, I've done something good for myself, and I feel more connected inside.

Movement/Dance

Movement in the form of a gentle to vigorous dance is greatly beneficial in assisting your body to stay in a peaceful state. It can be transforming. Some cultures have used movement and dance in their ceremonies. It can be a way to pray or to express and release emotions, and to connect with the inner core of our beings. Allow dance to assist your body to relax and release stress and tension. This can be a harmonious and a spiritual experience as you nurture yourself. Help yourself and your health by doing this form of body awareness to soothing music. Remember to breathe deeply as you glide your feet across the floor. Be creative and playful as you invite dance into your lifestyle, adding different types of music, singing, praising, or humming. The result is that music starts flowing naturally from you as someone who whistles or sings throughout your day.

Nature

Finding peace within is an essential ingredient to living and expressing a full life. One way to do this is to spend time in nature. Allow your bare feet to touch the grass or sand and receive the natural benefits from getting close to the earth. Wear natural fabric clothes such as cotton.

For people with high stress levels, taking time to lie outdoors for at least 5-10 minutes can be very beneficial. Lie face-up on a cotton sheet on the ground, observe the sky, and watch the clouds. Allow your mind to become still. Use a pillow for your head if needed. When you are ready, roll over and let your stomach area be nurtured in the same way by feeling the coolness or warmth from the earth. Allow your stress to melt away while you enjoy the great outdoors with nothing to distract you. Try it and notice the calming effect.

Sunshine

I am convinced that being in the sunshine for 5-10 minutes daily mid morning or late afternoon when possible has improved my vision. I originally followed this daily routine for two to three months and passed my driver's license eye exam for the first time since I was sixteen without my glasses.

While I'm outdoors in the sunshine or daylight, without wearing glasses or contacts, I do my eye exercises: I blink often to allow the contrast between sunlight and darkness to work my eye muscles. I roll my eyes from side to side and straight up and down, working muscles that normally only look straight ahead.

The sun is my daily small dose of sunshine vitamin, energizing me and providing a positive psychological calming affect.

Eating Habits

Help your health and digestive system by slowing down and taking approximately twenty minutes to eat each meal. Chew your food thoroughly until it becomes a mush, lubricated with saliva, making it easier to swallow and digest. Many times this extra chewing will eliminate belching, overeating, stomach pain, and indigestion, and help in losing or maintaining weight. Eating too fast tends to place more food in the system than the body requires. Help your body to be relaxed and be receptive for food rather than hurried, stressed, and tense.

Create a pretty place with silence or pleasant music for eating, and let your food be a blessing. Avoid clutter and loud noise that can affect your digestion. Be aware; taste and smell your food. Avoid automatic, routine meals. Slow down. Taste each bite as if it were your first time to eat that food. Ask yourself, "Do I enjoy this?" "Is it good for me?" "Could I eat better?" Make a commitment to honor your body more by feeding it nourishing food.

Purchase food that is in its natural form, unaltered by man's tampering or refining. Eat plenty of vegetables (raw and cooked) and fruits, along with whole grains such as wheat, rye, corn, oats, whole brown rice, legumes (dried beans), and dried fruits and nuts. Purchase organic food whenever possible; you can actually taste the difference in how the plants have been grown. Eat grilled, broiled or baked chicken, turkey, and fish.

If you are into juicing or buying fresh juice made at a health food store, you have probably already been convinced of the benefits. If you have never tried juicing, then try an experiment for 2-4 weeks. Purchase some fresh juice at your local health food store; carrot juice is a favorite. Start with small amounts until you acquire a taste for it. Drink a medium to large glass two to three times per week.

Drinking fresh juices is like giving your body superoctane gas. Fresh vegetables and fruit juices hardly require any digestion and are easily assimilated. Juices allow the body to have a nice rest, because it doesn't have to work so hard digesting and assimilating foods.

Once you are accustomed to fresh juices, you may want to buy the equipment to do juicing in your home. When buying equipment, look for a motor strong enough to grind carrots and beets. Some smaller motors will vibrate and walk across the counter top, spilling juice along the way.

Your local health food store will have a variety of books available on the benefits and combinations of juicing, including juice fasting.

When to Eat

Fuel the body at the beginning of the day by eating a wholesome breakfast. Allow three to four hours between meals. The stomach requires that time to digest food with its hydrochloric acid and then eliminate its contents. The stomach rests and then replenishes the hydrochloric acid as it awaits the next meal.

By continuous eating, the natural rhythm of proper food spacing, digestion, and elimination gets completely ignored. Don't snack between meals because the stomach never gets to empty thoroughly and ends up with both old and new food in the stomach. This can cause fatigue, indigestion, bloating, belching, and burning pain.

People with diabetes and low blood sugar have done very well on this program; if you have questions, please ask your doctor before making any changes.

Read Labels

Read product labels and become educated about the ingredients. The first ingredient listed represents the greatest percentage of the contents. If the first ingredient is water, sugar, or refined oil you may want to reconsider what you are buying and paying for. If the first ingredient is a fruit, vegetable, whole grain, beans, nuts or meat, you will know it has a higher nutritional value.

Other items to avoid:
* **Refined white sugar**, which is totally lacking in protein, vitamins and minerals.
* **Fructose**, like refined white sugar, is devoid of nutrients.
* **Refined cooking oil** is highly concentrated. It takes 12 to 15 cobs of corn to equal one tablespoon of oil, or 300 olives to equal 1/3 cup of olive oil. Concentrated refined oil lacks the ingredients found in nature needed to properly digest and assimilate the oil. Avoid deep-fried foods and those saturated with oils and grease.
* **Preservatives and additives:** a good rule of thumb is, if you can't pronounce it ask yourself if it has been derived from fruits, vegetables or nature. More often than not, it hasn't been.

Chose natural, fresh ingredients as often as possible and cut back or avoid processed foods and drinks that come in boxes and cans. Consider cold-pressed oil in moderation as an alternative to refined oil.

Fresh Water

Water makes up 65-75% of the body and is essential for optimum performance of the cell. Water flushes wastes and toxins through the urine and sweating. Thirst is not a reliable signal that your body needs water. Without adequate water we dehydrate.

Use your local library and health food store resources to determine what drinking, cooking, and bathing water is best in your area. You might want to have your water analyzed to give you accurate information. The sources of water available include mineral, distilled, filtered, spring, well or city water.

The amount of water your body should receive each day, in ounces, is your body weight divided by two.

Example: Weight of 150 pounds
150 divided by 2=75 oz., or nine 8-oz. glasses of water.

If you can't tolerate plain drinking water, add lemon or lime to enhance the taste.

It is best to space your water intake throughout the day and not drink one hour before or after meals. Drink a small amount (1/4 to 1/2 cup of fluid) with your meals to aid in the digestion of food but not enough to dilute the natural hydrochloric acid in the stomach. Stop drinking water two to three hours before bedtime to minimize getting up in the middle of the night and promote restful sleep.

Hunger pains can be a signal that the body needs water. Try drinking water the next time you feel hungry, and observe how you feel afterward.

Healthy urine should be clear like water and not have an odor. The darker the color and the stronger the smell of urine, generally the more toxic waste is placing a burden on the body without sufficient water to flush the system.

Body odor is a telltale sign of lack of water. Generally it is evident under the arms and in the breath and feet. Body sweating, including around the face and head, can indicate a lack of water and the system's being overworked and taxed.

An example of this is found in nature. If you were in the country and came upon a pond of water with little movement or no new water coming into it, you would probably be suspicious of the quality of the water. First the pond would start to evaporate, then to smell, and eventually it would become putrid.

Our bodies respond the same way. Without water we lower our energy as we dehydrate. We become toxic, sluggish, and exhausted.

Try water over caffeine, soft drinks, and alcohol. Your energy will naturally increase, and your body will thank you.

Fresh Air

Spend as much time as possible in the country to experience fresh air in nature. With plenty of fresh air and sunshine, perhaps doctors would be needed less often.

One would never think of eating food some other person had chewed, yet we breathe foul air over and over from having our homes and office buildings closed up. If you experience dust, fumes, animal hair, cigarette smoke or other odors, humidity, sore throats, sinus problems and allergies, an investment in a air cleaner that has been recommended by the American Lung Association can be very beneficial to you and your family's health.

Breathing, Lungs and Cigarettes

There are many programs and much information available on how to stop smoking. It's the addiction many seem to enjoy even if it is destroying their health. From everything else written, perhaps you will come up with ideas on your own of how to quit if you have a desire to do so. If you choose to continue smoking, you'll get the same results: coughing, lack of ability to smell, breath odor, tartar on teeth, polluted lungs, etc. The sacred self has great patience, but it lasts only so long until one day, when unexpectedly, your body breaks down. Don't wait for that to happen to you if you smoke. You may not get another chance to quit.

Breathing and the Organs

If a body organ was like your hand made into a fist, and you never moved that fist, whatever was inside would stay almost motionless. Our organs depend on body movement to enhance their function in the cleansing cycle. Very little body movement or shallow breathing hinders many systems and jeopardizes our vital organs and immune system because waste products don't get eliminated properly.

CHAPTER NINE

Other Helpful Remedies

My greatest teacher has been a two-year-old named Susan. Her mother, a massage client of mine, called me. Susan had been crying uncontrollably for five days. The doctors could not find anything wrong with her. Her mother brought her to me. I was in shock hearing such a small baby screaming hysterically, as though she was being tortured. The sound penetrated every fiber of my being. What could possibly be wrong? How could her parents have stood listening to her for five days?

I laid my hands on her back and head as her mother held her. I listened with my hands and did some hands-on work. After thirty minutes, Susan stopped screaming and released a very long, pleasant sigh. I could follow the sigh down through her body, watching it visibly shift. She smiled, started to breathe more deeply, and wanted to get down and play. I felt so blessed. I couldn't explain what happened, but I received a great inner wisdom of how it felt and sounded.

Susan slept in the same room with her parents, who were going through a divorce. She hadn't learned to talk in sentences, but she was taking in their emotional pain with no appropriate way to release it. Remembering the perfection of feeling in alignment, Susan had been screaming to go back to that place of perfection.

Susan helped me understand something that had happened to me years before. One day, after my face had healed and about two years after having regular massage therapy, my massage therapist utilized cranial work in our session. Suddenly my body shifted into a new way of being, one I hadn't known was possible. This brief taste of bliss lasted 5-10 minutes. I had a glimpse of what I had to look forward to.

The following remedies helped me get to that point, and can help you as well. These remedies require more "action" than those in the previous chapter, and may involve consulting with professionals.

Colon Care

The whole body can be affected by the condition of the colon. The colon, or large intestine, is an elimination system that also serves to hydrate the body. When it malfunctions, you are sometimes unaware of the cause and experience unexplained aches, pains, allergies, sinus problems, bad breath, indigestion, weight gain, bloating, constipation, cancer, etc.

Old, caked fecal matter makes it difficult for waste to pass through the body.

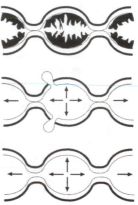

Over time blockages can create abnormal pouches or sacs called diverticula that can become inflamed.

An unobstructed colon allows waste matter to pass through the body quickly and easily.

Tension from emotional events is often stored in the solar plexus area of the body, through which the transverse colon passes. Unresolved tension affects all organs in that part of the body, particularly the colon. As the colon muscle tightens, constipation results. Proper colon care not only helps to bring the body back into balance, but can also release stored emotions.

A simple colon transit test can indicate how well your colon is functioning. This test measures the time it takes food to pass from your mouth through your digestive system and be eliminated from your body. Normal transit time should be from 18 to 24 hours.

Start the test in the evening. Eat nothing after the evening meal and wait three to four hours. Then eat one tablespoon of whole kernel corn, but don't chew it very well. Record the time. The corn will pass through the digestive system largely undigested. Watch for the undigested corn in your bowel movement and record the time. If the transit time is more than 24 hours, this may indicate your colon is not functioning normally and needs to be cleansed. Some people have gone three to six days before eliminating their corn. During that time the colon has become full of decayed waste, putrefying not only the colon but also affecting other areas of the body.

Educate yourself about your colon by reading books on colon cleansing. Visit your local health food store and investigate different fiber colon cleansers. Start with small amounts, noticing how you feel; too much too soon can result in gas, bloating, or constipation. Gradually increase to the recommended dosage, noticing any differences in the function of the colon.

Massaging your colon is also helpful. To do this, lie down on your back. Begin at the right side of your abdomen and end on your left. The left side, in the groin area, is where the colon ends, eliminating into the rectum. A healthy colon will be buoyant and flexible to touch and free of pain or discomfort. Usually discomfort or pain indicates impacted food. Massage these areas gently with the palm of your hand. (Walking is another way to massage your colon and encourage elimination through gravity and movement.)

Your bowel movements should be fibrous and not hard; you should not have to strain to eliminate. The fecal material should be fairly odor-free once toxic waste gets cleaned out of the colon. If this is not true for you, you may need to make some dietary changes. If you are constipated, you may need to drink more water. Start to eliminate white refined flour products, which have had the fiber stripped from them. White flour coats the lining of the colon similar to the way water and flour form a paste. Replace them with whole grains. Eat more fresh vegetables and fruit. They contain fiber, which acts like a broom, cleansing the lining of the colon and keeping it healthy.

If your colon transit time becomes a problem, consider seeing a colon therapist who has specific training in obstruction and disease of the colon, and who can treat you with professional colonics. A colonic is done with water gently traveling through the colon. The experience is usually gentle and the water is normally hardly felt because water enters and leaves the body using the natural flow of gravity. This process cleanses and removes old fecal matter, caked unhealthy particles, and mucus. Peristalsis, the colon's natural muscle contractions that move waste out of the body, improves. Cleaning the colon of years of old fecal build-up and toxic waste allows the colon to regain its normal tone.

Colon therapists will make suggestions as to how often to have your colon cleaned in this manner, depending on the results you have the first time. To find a local colonic specialist, look in the yellow pages of your phone book under "Colonic Irrigation" or "Health." Visit the office before scheduling an appointment; most colon therapists are professional, but you will want to make sure sanitation and hygiene are a priority.

If colon therapy is not available, or if you need extra support between visits, an enema using only water may be useful.

Once your colon is operating naturally, your energy will generally increase while pain and discomfort will decrease. You will not only improve your current health, but also possibly prevent future problems and maintain your weight more easily.

Friendly bacteria in the colon cause the breakdown and decomposition of the food you eat, causing proper elimination. These bacteria can get out of balance when we take medications or have diarrhea, upset stomach, illness, poor diet, acne, cold sores, or mouth ulcers.

Acidophilus is a product that can be found in health food stores in powder or capsule form. This is a natural, healthy bacteria culture that helps restore the colon's internal environment and proper balance. Taken as directed, results are sometimes noticed within 24 to 48 hours.

Why Massage Is Important

I personally believe in massage from my own years of experience. It has been very calming and beneficial in my recovering from trauma. I have taught massage students from all walks of life and observed the benefits of massage to their health as the class progressed. Massage techniques vary, but I always prefer the therapist who can "center" me the most, bringing my body to a state of calmness and relaxation. Once centered, all systems become more harmonized and increase the opportunity for healing.

Safe touch in itself is healing. Studies show that babies die if not touched, yet other babies stop crying who are gently given a back rub. As adults, we touch ourselves routinely while bathing. Massage allows our bodies to be given a nurturing touch, helps us connect to a deeper experience, and can be very soothing for people who have lived with mild to extreme stress.

Many techniques of massage are beneficial, including sports, relaxation, pain relief, injury, etc. Massage can be technical, mechanical, or spiritual; it depends on the therapist, whose intention, experience, and lifestyle are a big part of your massage experience. Therapists who don't take care of themselves give from their stress. Therapists who nurture themselves and practice the health principles they recommend to others will create a healing space for their clients. Spiritual massage therapists listen through their hands and other senses to become facilitators for healing.

Interviewing a therapist is perfectly acceptable before engaging him or her to do massage work on you. Explain what you want and where you feel pain. Once on the massage table, give the therapist feedback on whether you want more or less pressure from the touch. This is your session, and you are paying to have an ideal environment and experience.

Massage unwinds your stress and has a calming affect. It increases circulation and stimulates the lymph and immune system. It improves muscle tone and aids in digestion, reduces surgical recovery time, and improves mental and physical balance.

Massage has been around for more than 2,000 years. It has been used for prevention of illness, relaxation, relief of pain, and recovery from trauma and injury. It is not a luxury as much as a vital, natural healing therapy. The first few sessions take one to one and one-half hours, but the effect will last for two or three days. The body will do its own healing work with a little encouragement and facilitation from others. After having massage on a regular basis, most people are able to maintain the peaceful, relaxed harmony of their body for longer periods of time.

Massage can help you experience how much stress is in your body and how readily your body responds to removing the stress. A real self-love and appreciation happens when you notice your body becoming more flexible, healthier, and energized. This feeling of well-being happens for almost everyone, regardless of age.

Cranial Therapy

The head has 22 bones that are flexible and held together by a membrane. When we become tense from fear, trauma, and stress, these bones tighten. The adult human head weighs about eight pounds and pivots on the spine; watch most small children and notice their heads bobbing freely on their spines. Adult heads, on the other hand, demonstrate more stiff or rigid movement.

The cranial system interacts with the nervous system. Starting at the base of the neck, this is a fine network of electrical energy that goes throughout the body. When the cranial bones tighten, the head weighs the entire cranial system down, pushing directly on the central location where the nervous system begins and decreasing energy flow. A domino effect appears throughout the overall nervous system, possibly causing depression, fatigue, and lower energy. It is not obvious; it takes place subtly over time.

When the cranial bones are released through cranial therapy, the bones become flexible again. Chronic neck and shoulder pain disappears. The jaw, facial muscles, and back relax.

Cranial therapy helps access your own self-corrective healing processes. Almost everyone reports a deeper awakening spiritually, as well as greater emotional stability and self-worth.

There are a wide variety of therapies that include cranial work. The style of therapies can vary from a subtle, light touch to something more firm. Look for an individual with the style that works best for you and your needs.

Clothing, Color, and Personal Care Products

Natural fabrics like cotton, silk, linen, and wool will breathe with your body more naturally than others will. Choose fabrics, clothing and accessories that are soft to touch, perhaps even cuddly feeling.

Colors have been known to affect our moods. Break your routine; try wearing various new colors and notice the effect. Do you feel any different? There are books available on color therapy for clothing and decorating our homes and offices.

When purchasing make-up, shampoo, soap, etc., look at labels and choose natural ingredients. Check with your health food stores and local distributors that sell natural products, and try different brands until you find what works best for you.

Crisis Intervention

Being diagnosed with a chronic or even life-threatening condition is frightening and painful. Understanding the mechanics of the problem can be helpful, however. We become alerted to the urgency of our situation and are able to make informed decisions about what holistic direction to take.

The immune system, from my perspective, stands as a guardian over all functions of the body, ready to fight off anything that would invade or threaten its incredible intelligence for healing, harmony, and wholeness. This intelligence is in every cell and fiber of the body.

When symptom(s) appear, we tend to act as if all we need to do is gather them up and set them aside, and then we will immediately feel better. However, if we look deeper, the real problem is generally a weakened immune system that out-pictures itself visibly in the weakest area of the body. This produces symptoms labeled with names even the angels would have difficulty pronouncing! The label can feel condemning, shameful, and morally damaging. However, we can also see it as physical challenge from which we can learn.

Personally, I make every attempt to honor my God-given internal guardian and do everything I can to support its natural self-healing process in order to be restored. In this process the body's own intelligence can strengthen the area that has been weakened.

No matter how serious the situation appears to be, holistic remedies can help to bring the body into a state of balance. We can reach out to nature, reassured that natural prescriptions can assist us and complement whatever health program we are on.

Faced with such a diagnosis, begin to ask yourself questions:

1. Am I willing to take the time and effort to be with my condition, my weakened immune system, as if it were a sick child, loving it and nurturing it back to health?
2. Is medication what my body is lacking? The answer for me, obviously, was no.
3. If I have the weakened area cut out, will the problem truly go away?
4. If I were an immune system that was given large amounts of loving thoughts, would I mend faster? Yes! Love is still the greatest healer. The message of fear is the greatest destroyer. Every cell of your body responds to spoken or unspoken words and either become energized from positive reinforcement, or give up from fear.

There are many holistic alternatives available. You might be judged harshly by others when choosing this route. Choose wisely the individuals with whom you will share the path you have chosen. Stay open and trust yourself, and you will be guided.

The suggestions included in this chapter and "Daily Practice: 'Health' Yourself" can all be beneficial in your healing. Following are some additional suggestions for improving your immune system when you are faced with the diagnosis of a chronic or life-threatening condition:

1. Eliminate stress
2. Rest
3. Have colonics no less than once a month, more often if recommended by the colon therapist.
4. When juicing, the ideal juices are cold pressed and not exposed to heat from the speed of the juicer motor. This allows the juice to retain a maximum amount of its original vitamins and minerals.

5. Drink three to six eight-ounce glasses of fresh juice daily. The juice of organic carrots and green leafy vegetables are particularly high in minerals. Research which juices work best to assist your personal body needs.
6. Acknowledge that God is the ultimate physician and healer. Do your part to assist God's divine power of healing.
7. Even when the damage has gone so far that you see little or no improvement, continue to look for miracles.
8. Do all things in moderation, gentleness, and compassion, for the child within is ever ready to respond to love and to pleasantly surprise you.
9. Welcome your own discernment as to whether a medical, holistic, or combination program works best for your condition. Stay open and you will be guided.
10. When the time is right you will find yourself sharing with another in a similar situation that you have been in, and encouraging them. Just notice.

Additional Books and Reference Information

For additional information, check your local book stores, libraries or health food stores. Some health food stores and churches have directories of holistic classes, practitioners, therapists, recovery groups, and doctors. Also check local health magazines and newspapers. Your local yellow pages are also an excellent resource.

If possible, tour a health food store with the manager. Seek information. Look into herbs, sea salts for bath water, and aromatherapy oils as self-healing aids. Smell, feel, and listen to your own intuition. Take your time selecting what to buy. On occasion some salespeople will try to convince you that you need a health program of vitamins, etc., that you may not need or be able to afford. Respect their suggestions, but follow your own clear thinking.

CHAPTER TEN

Measure Your Joy

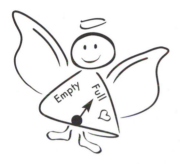

I have found that there are two ways to make a decision or take action in life. One is to go blindly ahead on others' recommendations and learn by hard experiences, disliking some of your results. Have you ever said, "I knew better than to do that . . . ." Or, "I did that only to please someone else and I felt miserable" or, "I don't know what I feel, so I'll follow others"?

The other is to follow the guidance of your own spirit, being confident and enjoying the results you get. Affirm your own clear thinking by learning to trust your own intuition to say "yes" and "no." "I trusted myself to make my own decision about...and it feels right."

Measure Your Joy is a daily exercise in distinguishing the difference between these two methods and encouraging you to trust your own God-given Spirit to lead you to more joy.

Measurement Guide

When making decisions about your daily life from telephone calls, invitations, and your daily schedule to significant relationships, family, friends, co-workers, etc., the **Joy Measurement Guide** can help you become aware of your body language and energy as a way to promote your health and happiness.

This is not a test; there are no right or wrong answers. **Measure Your Joy** is an awakening to how you live and the results you get. Become an observer as you get clarity about how you do what you do. Perhaps you will want to congratulate yourself for progress with your mental and physical health, or you may become aware of how you lower your energy and your self-esteem. Once you notice the differences, you can make the necessary changes from a desire for greater fulfillment and joy.

Review this chapter daily and weekly for as long as it takes to live the life you desire. Practice measuring your joy by:

* Reviewing the measurement scale (one is less joy, ten is greater joy) and the descriptions that follow.
* Determining where on the scale you find yourself living most often.

Later in this chapter you will get to review the results that will possibly have a profound, positive impact on your daily experience.

Measure Your Joy Scale

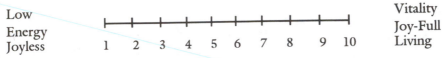

Low Energy Joyless   1 2 3 4 5 6 7 8 9 10   Vitality Joy-Full Living

Rate Your Decision

One to Four
Unfortunately, this is where many of us have lived our lives.

* Brings me no joy. I might even resent thinking about doing it. I'll do it, but it doesn't make me feel good.
* I feel like I'm being used.
* I deny my own needs and sacrifice myself for others.
* I've done it before; I'm not motivated. I'll do it for them!
* My heart's not in it; I'll do it only for the money!
* I don't know what I feel or want.

Five
The start of self-realization and taking responsibility

* I'm more aware, I start to notice my body language and energy.
* I choose not to rescue others and violate my energy, time or space.
* I question doing it; overall I'm not feeling good about whatever...
* I can decide it's not for me to do or I can get someone else to do it.
* I'm group minded and know that I'm doing it out of unconditional love—I make an intelligent decision and will bear the discomfort of my actions.

Six to Nine
Life is good! I've gone too far to turn back.

* This feels better, fits my personality more.
* I'm in tune with my energy and pace myself.
* I define my boundaries, choosing peace within and out.
* I have positive thoughts and conversations.
* My joy is to rest right now and take action later.
* This has my interest, is highly creative, and brings me fulfillment.

* I feel pleased, proud of my activities.
* Time goes by faster, I enjoy my days.
* I have goals for myself.
* I've learned to say honestly "yes" and "no."
* I have rewards for myself for doing something well.

Ten

My wisdom comes through my life experiences. I celebrate the endless possibilities that await me, regardless of my age or situation.

* I feel joy, excitement, and love doing it, even if I don't get paid.
* I notice increased happiness and health when I'm having fun.
* I notice money isn't an issue; I start having abundance.
* I live one day at a time and define that day.
* I ask for what I want and need, and make healthier decisions.

Notice Your Daily Living Results

As you choose activities using the Joy Measurement Guide, you will see improved results in your daily life. Be gentle with yourself as you make improvements. Hopefully you'll be proud of your progress, reminding yourself that you have a lifetime of starting each and every day brand new. Based on the Joy Measurement Guide, following are the results we can expect from the choices we make:

One to Four

* Lower self-esteem, drained energy, pain or illness, loneliness or depression
* Self-abusive behavior, increased addictions
* Expression of fear and anger
* Going through life acting like you don't care
* Finding fault with self and others

Five

* Awakening to healthier more positive choices and proudly welcoming the results in the body and in life.

Six to Ten

* More physical energy, self-love, and appreciation.
* Increased happy heart experiences.
* Sense of pride in integrity towards myself and values.
* Being true to self
* Accepting myself as God's creation, loving my defects and shortcomings.

For example: You're working on a project that has excited you, but you feel your energy beginning to wane. You feel tired and want to take a break, but you're concerned about how your boss will feel about it.

Having learned from the Joy Measurement Guide, you begin to get quiet. You ask yourself, "What should I do?"

Perhaps you notice that on a scale of one to ten, your joy in the project has dropped from an eight to a three. Your old behavior pattern would have been to be loyal to the project and to push through your exhaustion, leaving you feeling resentful and self-betrayed, and perhaps with body aches or other symptoms.

Instead, you decide to take that needed break and begin to relax. Your body responds to the tender care you insist on giving it, and you feel your energy begin to expand. Your mind begins to rest. When you are ready, you return to the project, this time with self-appreciation and vitality. Refreshed, you complete the project easily.

Taking care of yourself might have felt a little risky at first, but you acknowledge those feelings and trust yourself. As you welcome this new learned behavior, you set an example for others, including your boss.

Having a joy-filled life may take days or years to learn. Be gentle with yourself. Joy will bring you the greatest satisfaction. It's not a false high from the abusive behavior of drugs, alcohol or other addictions that ultimately leave the soul empty. Measuring Your Joy is about connecting with your own God-given spirit, which has individual likes and dislikes.

The following is an affirmation you may want to repeat during your daily routine:

"I'm rewarded with an abundance of every good thing as I'm true to, and follow my God-given spirit in joy."

CHAPTER ELEVEN

Faster Recovery Time

Some people, myself included, can be extremely sensitive to statements and actions that other people would overlook. Our minds have been in fight or flight, compounded by the stress and fear of the possibility of a terminal conditions or threats of deforming. We may feel "on edge," vulnerable, and insecure. Therefore we may strive to guard and protect ourselves because of our desire to accelerate our own healing and not have setbacks. While we may respond to dangerous or life-threatening attacks well, we find that the "little things" get to us.

Even years after physical healing or removal from a traumatic situation we can have automatic emotional responses to small everyday events that can be devastating, humiliating, overwhelming, panicking, or confusing. Minor accidents, making a mistake, and encounters with inconsiderate people can create emotional stress that can last for hours, during which time most of us haven't known how to explain our reactions, let alone figure out a solution. We react, feeling as if someone threatened our lives. It is hard to feel secure and trust life not knowing how we may react the next time.

An Old Way of Responding

1. The Event
For example, someone or something surprises us and takes us off guard. We may get emotional and feel insulted, fearful, shocked, or angry. Reactions may be mild to extreme.

2. Our mind races about what he said, I said, she did, I should have done, etc. We may say to ourselves:
* Why was I left out?
* Just like me! I'm so clumsy or forgetful.
* They treat me different than other people!
* You just don't understand me!
* How dare they!

* I did it wrong! I am wrong!
* It is my fault.

We react from self-defense. We may throw a tantrum, verbalize angry words, or start whining and complaining, insisting the other person is wrong, or we turn the anger on to ourselves. We feel shame or blame about our reacting instead of responding appropriately. We worry about what the other person thinks, judging ourselves as right or wrong.

If we're not verbal we may become speechless, internalize our anger, numb out and let the other person have their way, all because we can't think clearly in the moment of distress. We end up feeling like a weakling with no words to defend or express our feelings. We can't verbally express ourselves but soon our minds ramble with explosive self talk.

3. Physical Responses

Our body responds to the stress with physical symptoms, which may include tension, weakness, trembling, pressure, chest pain, dizziness, or shortness of breath.

On an emotional level we may experience depression, overwhelm, mood swings, sleeplessness, fatigue, or shallow breathing.

Illness can follow. We may experience body pain, sore throat, stomach or headaches, cough or cold, or sinus attacks.

The longer the turmoil and brooding over our insecure thoughts continues, the stronger the feelings and sensations build and last. We can hang on to these types of irritations for hours, days and even weeks.

The more informed and healed we become, the more we will notice a decrease in symptoms and faster recovery time.

A New Way to Respond

Recovery begins the moment we are willing to slow down and notice our behavior.

1. The same event happens

We become aware that we are feeling shock, frightened, and emotional. We remind ourselves that we are okay, safe, and capable of taking immediate care of ourselves.

Stop! Everything else can wait. We sit down long enough to release our emotions so we can regain our composure and clear thinking. Now we can sort through healthy steps to regain a peaceful state of being.

2.   Take charge of your thoughts

We begin to take charge of our thoughts. Taking control of our thoughts the moment they start to ramble and explode can dispose of many of our temperamental upheavals.

3.   Make sense of it all

Make sense of it all by journaling or finding someone to listen to us as we release and express our feelings.

Talking and emotional release reduce or eliminate body symptoms of lowered energy and illness. There is a difference between just reporting our feelings through talk and experiencing them physiologically as we express. Speaking out about our feelings, even if it feels uncomfortable, releases the internal, erupting, emotional stress that normally would have caused our body symptoms. We can appraise the situation and gain clarity, bringing calmness and relief, avoiding the sacrificing of our inner and outer peace.

Other people usually don't get upset about how we feel unless we start blaming them, so we can use words wisely: "When you did that, this is how I felt (frightened)." "This is how it affected me (my breathing became uncomfortable and I felt pain in my chest)."

We can choose not to lash out in rage that can cause tension and increase symptoms or disorders. Rage is defensive: "Why do I always have to be the one to change?" Feelings and thoughts cannot be reported objectively in the heat of a disagreement.

4.   Get physically involved in something more enjoyable.

As soon as possible, take action. Walking or physical movement is helpful in assisting our bodies to relax. Focus on something positive, redirecting the body, mind, and energy.

5.   Acknowledge your improvements, no matter how small.

It is helpful to continually strive to validate ourselves for any and all new awareness. Practice over and over until you have developed a healthier way of responding, and releasing these fearful events.

6.   Notice insights about your reactions:

* Thoughts hook into our feelings, making them better or worse.
* Feelings intensify or decrease, depending on our thoughts and actions following the incident. When we release our feelings by utilizing the "Natural Healing Process" (chapter seven), our racing thoughts slow down.

* This has my interest, is highly creative, and brings me fulfillment.
* I feel pleased, proud of my activities.
* Time goes by faster, I enjoy my day.
* Our reactions are generally based on experiences from our past.

We may not be able to always control our feelings and emotional responses to the little things in life. It is not helpful to deny them, but following the reaction we can change our thoughts.

7. Communicate, clarify, and evaluate

We can choose to be willing to drop our emotional judgements, impatience, and irritations and be willing to communicate. When we have doubts, we can check them out. It is worth all the effort it takes to learn how to communicate, asking for what we need and want and choosing not to stuff our emotional pain or to feel embarrassed about what others might think of us.

We can evaluate the fact that most of our reactions tie into our wounded past and continue to appear emotionally as real danger or threats, when in reality they are not.

8. Look at the odds

Little things in life will happen. Be willing to accept them with confidence, perhaps even humor, and not as a victim.

9. Approach these events with compassion

Long-lasting recovery, self-esteem, and empowerment happen when we can see the situation from another's perspective (which at the time of the event may be impossible). Putting ourselves in another's place, with their background and their emotional pain, can be insightful. Become aware that people can have bad days and act rudely. They can be impatient, unkind, harsh, and inconsiderate because they have stress, are lonely, or have troubled hearts. It is more average than rare. It is not about you.

We realize that we really don't know peoples' backgrounds and their fear of success or failure. Are they healthy or sick, lonely or happy, calm or fearful? We all share the need to feel accepted, loved, rested, and secure and to have compassionate people in our lives.

When we are able to see a situation in this way, we are less likely to blame ourselves. We give up being self-critical and instead practice self-appreciation, which in turn can improve our health.

Gaining understanding about our reactions and developing healthier ways to respond are the keys to mental and emotional health, which can lead to more positive encounters with others along life's journey.

CHAPTER TWELVE

How To Write Your History

You will know when the time is right to start on this exercise. You may begin to want to understand your past, the journey that got you to this point in life. You may become curious about your patterns in relationships, careers, and illnesses that repeat themselves.

This is also a great exercise for those people who have miracle healing stories about what God has done in their lives, and who may have a burning desire to share those stories to encourage others and offer hope. This may get you motivated.

Writing your history is very revealing. It can be very emotional, yet healing and rewarding. Every time you say, "That is all there is to remember about this event," more information will come to you. Be patient, and stay curious and open.

If you recall from "Healing Takes Whatever It Takes," I discovered that even after the physical healing, I was carrying my past with me. Writing helped me review my patterns visually on paper. There is an old saying: "You can't solve something unless you know what it is."

I found it very helpful to have several kinds of therapy or group support available to encourage my efforts in healing certain areas of my past as I wrote.

Preparation

Remind yourself often that you are not doing this to relive the past or to get stuck once more in the pain of the memories. This process is to acknowledge how you developed your beliefs and patterns of behavior. It is about affirming yourself for all you have been through. It is about forgiveness and healing. You are rewarding yourself by making decisions about what you want to believe, how you want to live, and how you want to treat yourself and be treated by others. This is about you and your future.

See yourself as a child who could have grown up in many different families, taking on the individual beliefs and patterns of behavior of each of them. How would your life have been growing up in a wealthy family, middle class or poor? How different would it have been in a stable, healthy, supportive family?

Choose to write, dream, affirm yourself, set aside your hurtful beliefs and patterns, and make healthy decisions about the "child" within.

How to Start

Get a journal or spiral notebook, or whatever feels appropriate. Begin by writing your earliest memories, every one of them. Allow an extra blank page(s) in between each memory for additional thoughts. Try to list your memories in chronological order. If you have have limited or nonexistent memories of your childhood, start with what you do remember and go forward. Those lost years may or may not be revealed later. Don't rush this process. It might take a couple of years to cover your entire life, so pace yourself. Even the smallest event will end up having more details as you do the exercise.

You might be surprised at how emotional you still feel over something that happened long ago. Unexpressed emotions may still feel very intense. Take notice: **these painful emotions are revealing themselves because it is time to stop ignoring and denying them, and to begin healing and releasing them.** You may need to rewrite the memories over and over or even discuss them with someone. By acknowledging them now, you support your mental, emotional, spiritual, and physical well-being.

Another step to writing your history is to ask yourself some questions, using a different colored pen or pencil to record your answers. You can choose whether to take this step while writing your history, or wait until you have finished it. Use the following questions as a guide, but be willing to make up your own questions as well.

1. **"What belief did I get from this memory?"**
    * About myself
    * About others
    * About God
    * About life
    * About authority figures

2. **"How did this memory or event make me feel?"**
    * Sad, happy, mad, lonely, quiet, embarrassed, weak, strong, big or small, etc.

Examples:

* This event made me feel proud and built my self-esteem. I could share my feelings; I was heard. I could trust being myself in making choices. I stayed healthy, alert and energized.
* This event was very hurtful. I stopped trusting and withdrew. I started believing something was wrong with me because I was treated this way. I got ill and depressed.

3. **"Are there similar characteristics between people I know now and those from my past?"**

   * Finding these common threads can show you what needs to be healed, or perhaps what you can celebrate!

4. **"When I need comfort or want to numb out, what do I do?"**

   * I spend money, or crave food, chocolate or alcohol when I'm angry, emotional, depressed or stressed, etc.

5. **"How many hours, months, or years of my life have I felt creative, artistic, highly motivated, playful, fulfilled, and inspired?**

   * Highlight these, because they might be significant when you are exploring a new lifestyle.

You will see the negative beliefs and patterns that you learned. They trick us into believing that we are who **they** are. Acknowledge your past, and learn from it. Determine very clearly what healthy beliefs you'll want to keep and add to them. Make decisions about getting therapy if you need it; having supportive people around you will help you make self-improvements.

After writing your history, you might consider making a written commitment as a way to summarize your past and make decisions about your future. It might go something like this:

"I dedicate this commitment to the one I love and care about—the one I look at in the mirror every day, the one who walks and talks with me, the one who will be with me when the clouds open up and I leave my friends and family behind.

"I know that every day I can choose how I will act and react, and what I will believe about myself and others. I am now attracted to positive, uplifting, successful people and opportunities. I now commit my life and spiritual well being, to be guided to my purpose and passion—that which will bring me joy, will also keep me healthy and happy. I am now directed away from all hurtful people, thoughts and events. I give thanks, forgive, and let go of my past.

"My mental health, happiness and peaceful spirit are my greatest blessings, I will protect and honor them. I give thanks that I'm alive and have choices."

Date_____ Name_____

After writing your history you may want to incorporate the ideas in the chapter "Measure Your Joy" as a way to begin your future.

CHAPTER THIRTEEN

To Imagine Is To Believe

Through the power of the imagination, we impress upon the body the concepts we hold in the mind. I can imagine I have some awful condition, and through my own thoughts send messages that can manifest or worsen the condition. On the other hand, I can improve my health through the same process, sending positive messages through healthy thoughts.

The imagination is interesting. If you want a red car but have never seen one, it becomes harder to believe that you could own one. Yet the imagination has been used for centuries by athletes to rehearse before a performance the exact results they want to achieve. Using the same concept for healing is no different.

For example, if I have a liver problem but know nothing about the function or location of the liver, my mind is left to imagine and even exaggerate the condition, all based on fear. Fear is very deadly, as the mind will follow the directions of the unspoken or spoken word.

Instead, I can get correct information about the liver, locate the area in my body, and start visualizing healing energy taking place. I can do this in a variety of creative ways. I can draw mental pictures of what I want the end results to look like. I even can create images of little helpers; mine are angels carrying healing love energy in the form of a warm, soft, flowing rainbow of colors that nurture every cell, transforming them back to health. I can visualize sending love into the area and expand out into other areas, removing any dysfunction. In my mind I can see the word "love" written on an area of my body that is hurting. My sacred self identifies with love, even if I'm in too much pain to feel or believe it. There are no specified ways to use your imagination other than doing it in love and creativity, moving out of fear into compassion. If the diseased area doesn't heal completely or respond, I believe love still can have a profound effect on the mind and body.

I believe that in the future more people will turn to imagination and visualization. They will prove to themselves the power of the mind when used correctly for their highest good. This is another form of prayer. God spoke and creation happened. I believe God imagined it first.

How fast would our imaginations work if we won a lottery? With new possibilities of everything we longed for now available, we would spend the money over and over in our minds, enjoying every moment. The excitement alone of having won could possibly heal a serious ailment, even before having the money in hand. Think about it: if this could be possible, then perhaps the greatest remedy is **joy, joy, joy** by creating a positive, healthy attitude and uplifting lifestyle. I think it would be fun to overdose on joy. Unfortunately, many of us have done it on fear and worry, or sought the false high from drugs or alcohol.

I met a man who could measure cancer cells in a patient and do a one-hour visualization using his imagination, sending love into the blood. One hour later, the patient had fewer cancer cells.

I have a special friend, whose birth name means "Fair One." He is in his sixties and had an artificial artery put in his leg. After he came home from the hospital, I went to visit with him. The doctor had used metal staples or clamps to close the incision up and down his leg. The skin was bright, shining red, and stretched from being extremely swollen. It was hot and feverish. There was no use in trying to touch it or do any type of massage, so I started singing to him and doing visualizations, using his own mind to see energy flowing freely from his head to his feet and balancing itself. We traveled with the mind from the foot to the knee to the waist to the head, then down the back to the hips to the feet. Then we imagined seeing swirls of energy going from side to side and expanding. One hour later the swelling went down visibly, the redness lightened, and within hours his leg was fairly normal in size. The God-given mind had helped circulate his energy through an inflamed area and calmed his leg.

It is an honor knowing him; he gave me the name of "Wind Spirit," claiming I touch people's lives with visible and invisible love. I feel honored for the many experiences such as this that I have had and the privilege of facilitating healing in others.

Another friend was in the hospital awaiting back surgery. The doctors had her on maximum pain medication, but it wasn't enough. I brought my guitar and sang to her and started to imagine her angels, who absorbed and removed her pain while she rested in their arms. Soon afterward she was more relaxed, and the pain had decreased.

We need only dare to be creative and start telling stories that address the situation in a loving, supportive tone of voice and confidence that what we visualize becomes reality.

Negative Use of Imagination

If we don't understand the mechanics of how imagination works, we can use it in devious and harmful ways. For example, you're dashing around the house getting ready to leave. The phone rings, and you pick it up. It's your talkative friend, Gabby, who has no respect for your time or if the call is an inconvenience to you. You tell her you need to leave. Gabby informs you it won't take long and insists that you attend a party she's planning. She needs an answer tonight because she has to make reservations. Gabby urges, "Please say you'll come."

Without checking with yourself, you blurt out the words, "Okay, I'll go," just to get rid of her. When you hang up, you are furious with Gabby, but also angry with yourself. One more time you got suckered in. You feel powerless to tell her you really don't want to spend an evening with those people. "Why didn't I say no?" you ask yourself. "I wish there was some way I could get out of it! I wish I could think up an excuse for not going tomorrow night!" You're miserable and continue to chastise yourself for agreeing, but know you'll somehow force yourself to go in order to keep your good word.

The next morning you awaken, and your body language starts to tell the truth. Your sacred self has started rebelling; you now have a terrible headache and sore throat. You pop some pills; you gargle, pace the floor, go to bed. The misery increases. Finally you pick up the phone. "Gabby, I'm very sick and won't be able to go to your party tonight. I'm so sorry because I was looking forward to being with your friends. Love you, goodbye." You hang up the phone, breathe a big sigh, and toss a bunch of newspapers up in the air as a way to show your relief. Soon afterwards, you notice your headache has gone and the sore throat is disappearing.

We've all done this time and time again, beginning as children. How many of us got sick just before going to school, but felt better once we got to stay home? Our faithful body doesn't lie; our imagination and minds are to be respected as dear friends whom we don't want to violate. We slowly learn to protect the space inside and outside that our divine vessel lives in while our soul waits patiently.

Fantasize a Rare Invention

Once upon a time new technology was developed to create a robot whose body was made from the finest, rarest materials, sculpted and shaped to have the perfect resemblance of a human body, with the greatest smile painted on its pretty face. People were excited that this robot would revolutionize our futures.

It was highly sophisticated for our day and time. It showed up every day wearing the latest designer wardrobes of fashionable robot suits. It was highly efficient and reliable, and could perform hundreds of tasks.

The shock of this amazing invention eventually wore off, though, and the robot went unnoticed by others as it did everything from washing clothes to making sales calls. Ingenious, it automatically completed every assignment without a sense of smell, taste, hearing, or needing to take a break.

After many years of service, one day the friendly robot wore out. It suddenly fell over and stopped. Experts were called in to examine this faithful servant. Ever so slowly they dismantled its armor to get to the heart of why it stopped. Upon looking inside, some speculated they would find a hidden, exclusive treasure for future generations: the secret to creating more robots that wouldn't break down.

Upon delving deeper for the treasure, what do you think they discovered? The robot wasn't a "what" after all. "Who" do you think they discovered? Listen, and you'll recognize the voice coming from within that armor, calling for help. Get quiet and listen to the tone of the voice. Is it a teenager or an adult? Begin to look for resemblances. You'll know them well when they step out of that fancy suit.

We label this reality of fruitless work and emptiness an addiction, while our best friends and families are often too busy to notice us walking around in joy-less bodies, having lost the passion for life, depressed, lonely, running on empty, and molded to belong in society—lost in a robot suit.

The above describes my story of losing myself at home and in the office. The voice that stepped out of that robot suit many years ago was very faint and weak. Over time I have been resurrected to live in a body I enjoy and marvel at, and through the process have discovered more of my authentic purpose in life. As a storyteller, I use this story when I'm with people who understand this scenario all too well and are choosing to become free.

Perhaps this story hits some similar notes for you or someone you know. It is time to recognize our patterns and help each other break out of our own armor before we break down. Then, and only then, can we be spiritually set free.

Our soul's plea is for us to live our purpose and passion, the "real treasure," and to live in fragments of love no longer. May our prayer be, "Lord, deliver me to my passion" so we can go to bed at night saying, "Thank you, God, for this incredible day."

Rich blessings. Happy treasure hunting!

Imagination and Spoken Words

What is the difference from ordinary thoughts and words spoken or heard everyday from those spoken during prayer? We create fear or love daily in our lives by the images we place in our minds. Believe only good is coming out of your prayers, words, and actions. Explore possible end results; imagine events and situations having happy endings. The mind and imagination are very suggestive. What we see and hear stays with us, and what is negative acts like a toxic poison. I can't put poison in and believe that after awhile it won't matter, that "it's just a movie." Relish and choose more the sacred use of your imagination. As your body needs nutritious foods, so does your soul hunger for love, peace, joy, beauty, playfulness, and harmony as spiritual food.

To imagine it is to start believing it.

CHAPTER FOURTEEN

Heal By Expressing and Connecting

If you consider yourself happy and healthy, feel complete and full of love, and your life is filled with joy as you create your life's purpose, you may want to skip over reading this chapter and go to the next one.

Help is on its way, however, if you experience emotions as tangible energy that is interrupting your happiness. This is for those times when life appears stuck or feels very hard, perhaps even unfair, when feelings are bubbling up inside and your mind rambles continuously, or when you may be having physical or emotional pain.

I don't believe there are enough pain killers, surgeries, drugs, addictions, or alcohol to squelch the various cries of emotional pain, negative body memories, and spiritual emptiness. When they start erupting, they demand attention. We can numb them for awhile, but they will eventually resurface bigger and louder than ever. Admitting the problem and taking appropriate loving action is the wise and healthy answer toward finding a solution.

The importance of healing emotionally was brought home to me in a poignant way. A dear friend, who taught alternative medicine and holistic health to hundreds of people, got cancer. In our last conversation before she died I asked, "What do you think caused you to get cancer?"

Holding my hands, she looked into my eyes and with all sincerity said, "Georgie, my last few years have been so lonely. I'm no longer able to teach, and my retirement home is too far away from my students for them to visit. If I could have had people like yourself around me all along the way, sharing our talents, emotions, and wisdom, I don't think I would have gotten cancer." I sang at her funeral, knowing only too well how her ending in life could have been mine.

My emotional healing took time and went through many stages. As you review my list, notice which have been true for you:

1. **Denial**
    * The first year I kept my condition a secret, telling everyone there was nothing seriously wrong with me.

2. **Shield of Armor**
    * God gave me extra strength to endure and have persistence.

3. **Angry Avoidance**
    * I kept busy. Everything I did had to be done NOW!

4. **Temporary Truth**
    * I promised God that if I got healed, I would evangelize, getting others to believe. I was begging in desperation, wanting to believe in God myself.

5. **Depression**
    * I couldn't support myself financially any longer than a day or week at a time. I was unable to read a book, drive, or dream about creating my future and what I could make out of my life. I felt hopeless and even looked it!

6. **Grieving**
    * Eventually I was able to start releasing my pent-up emotions and deep inner pain.

7. **Truth**
    * I reclaimed by dignity and spirituality. My emotional pain and fear began to release, with peace, love, and joy taking their place.

8. **Traumatic Body Memories**
    * These were impregnated in every cell of my body. Transforming, healing, and rejuvenating them took time.

The self-help exercises given in this chapter helped me become healthier. They include solutions I found when I was isolated and therapy wasn't financially feasible or readily available, although you can use them as a complement to professional therapy as well. I suggest that you read the entire chapter before beginning. Take what fits as your own remedies. Add to them or leave some for later, maybe even years later. Do them from a longing to be connected and filled with greater understanding, self-love, and appreciation. These do come after time; they are your birthright.

When doing some of these exercises, you may feel the tears begin to come. Crying is most helpful when you can do it with another, creating a safe space in which to grieve. Many of us hide our emotions from others and only show them our false smiles. Crying is healing. It is being real with ourselves and those significant, supportive people who can open up to more of their own truth from our example.

The period of time after each self-help exercise is very significant; it is as important or even more so towards encouraging further healing. Don't cut your time short. Review the chapter "Daily Practice: 'Health' Yourself" for ideas on nurturing yourself after completing an exercise.

Once an exercise has been completed, leave it behind you. Don't think about it any longer. Do something playful and healthy, or continue to rest.

Exercise 1 - Write, Write, and Write
Use when feeling frustrated or overwhelmed and seeking change.

This exercise may take some time, so find a comfortable place and put on some soothing music. You will need a note pad or several pages of writing paper and your favorite pen. Remember to breathe deeply throughout this exercise.

Start to write out all your thoughts and feelings on paper. Don't read what you write, just write as fast as you can. Don't try to think about spelling, grammar, or doing it right. If you can't think of something to write, write about not being able to think; eventually the feelings will surface.

If the mind gives you messages that tell you, "I don't know how to write," then doodle, but fast and with large expressive motion and no judgment; just keep the pen flowing. The feelings will eventually give you messages in the form of words to write.

Crying is a great healer, so don't stuff the tears that might come. Cry and write. Write big. Talk and write—but write. Write the inner unspoken words of your soul. Write about what is bothering you.

What eventually happens after many pages is that the mind becomes calm. You begin to have clarity of thought, and perhaps even some "ah-has!" Note gradual increases of energy as you "help yourself be heard."

The important next step is to release your writing by letting go, without reading what you wrote. Here are several methods I have found helpful. You may find better ones that are even more creative for you.

Holding your papers in both hands, say this blessing or prayer, or create your own:

"I am forgiven and I forgive others; we've each done the best we knew how at any given moment. May I open now to my healing.

I'm on a new path and have gone too far to turn back. I will seek more joy and let go of fear. The God of creation, who is my creator, now teaches me how I can have more self-love and appreciation. I ask believing that this same creator will lead me to greater spirituality and inner wisdom. My spirit is being filled. However long it takes to fill my vessel, I will respect the process of my own healing."

Then rip the written pages up in small pieces, blessing their release. Burn them in the fireplace, put them in the garbage dumpster, or bury them in the back yard or a sacred place outdoors.

This exercise gets the stressful events, conditions, and people out of your system in a healthy, safe way. You can write on a computer, although for me there is something rewarding, and more healing, about writing by hand. Taking the time to take this journey and listen to the story behind the dysfunction of our lives creates increased knowledge, growth, health, and happiness. Eventually, the dysfunctions we have will no longer paralyze us.

If you need help, be willing to reach out for the therapies and people who can help you go deeper into yourself and come out energized. I don't deliberately dig into my past memories unless they are causing me pain or discomfort. Trust the process; you'll know when it's time. Low energy is a sure sign it's time to dig again.

Exercise 2 - Turning Anger Inside Out
Use when feeling disgusted, outraged, and angry, and when life appears unfair, or when the body feels low on energy.

There are many reasons for feeling angry; there are even more reasons to want anger to heal and not destroy us. We feel anger when we violate ourselves or allow someone to violate our space or lives.

Angry feelings short-circuit our lives and cut us off from our joy. It is very important not to deny anger, but to have a safe avenue to vent the pent-up feelings. Anger held inside turns into aches, pains, illness, and worse, so if it becomes real in your life, take these preventive measures to release the anger.

Healing unexpressed anger is very safe and rewarding. Anger is good. It pushes our buttons until we take a look at our lives and what we want to be different. This exercise will bring you increased clarity as well as physical benefits such as deeper, freer breathing and prevention of illness.

Find a room where you won't be disturbed, preferably when you're at home alone. Gather up a pile of newspapers and a large garbage bag. Sit in a comfortable position, with or without music. Sometimes it is better just to be alone with your emotions, thoughts, and feelings in the quiet; you decide what works best. Breathe often; breathe deeply.

Start by ripping those newspapers into small pieces, tearing chunks and layers of papers at a time and putting words with each rip. As you continue you will work up a sweat, which verifies the process is working—you're releasing the anger along with the thoughts and feelings connected to it. Make angry sounds if you can do this without family or neighbors getting involved.

When you sweat and take your anger out on the papers, you'll start to breathe more freely and feel calmer, and perhaps even smile. It feels good. It is freeing. Rip until you need to rest. Stop when you feel you've accomplished getting out that stuff that has been poisoning your goodness. Do it as often as you need to.

When you are done, gather your pile of shredded paper. Place it in a garbage bag and tie it tightly at the top. Toss it in the garbage or dumpster, preferably outside.

If you need additional help after this exercise, remember that it is just a telephone call away. Everywhere there are support groups, therapy groups, churches, recovery meetings, even free city services. Having one individual with you while you express, however, is the most optimum experience. Don't stop asking until you get the help you want and need.

Exercise 3 - Believe and Let Go
Goal Setting

Getting answers to prayers or requests can be rewarding. One way to satisfy the longing for fulfillment is to enhance your belief system with a sacred ritual. I suggest you keep this ritual private between you and your God.

You'll need a small box that is big enough to hold a week's or month's worth of requests. You will also need paper and pen. Create a personal place to store your box, but where you can go to it often.

Give yourself permission to play and be creative as you decorate your box. You can add stickers, paste some of your favorite pictures from magazines or your favorite snapshots, gift wrap it, or whatever else comes to mind. Cut a slit in it through which to insert your requests. You might want to name the box My God Box, My Joy Box, My Angel Box, My

Answer Box, or whatever other name is meaningful to you. By adding candles and pictures of Jesus, Mary, or your favorite saint(s) or teacher(s), and/or angel figurines and statues of saints, you can create your own altar.

This is a great exercise for receiving answers and letting go. This exercise is not about trying to control your situation. It's about building trust in prayers and divine guidance. You can add the following words to your request: "this or something better. Your will be done."

Goals Go in the Box

Sit comfortably and quietly. Write your goals, requests, and prayers; what would you like to see happen today, this week, or this month? Include any subject such as health, relationships, career, housing, travel, finances, etc. The greatest thing about active dreaming is not the goal itself as much as what going after a goal does for you. Creating keeps us alive, not buried alive.

Successful businesses do this often. They call it goal setting with an action plan, which includes positive thinking, imagination, and focused action in order to accomplish the goal.

Write with faith that your innermost thoughts are being heard and answered, that this or something better is coming your way. Don't beg; rather, write starting with "I want. . . . I'm open and ready for these good things or better to happen." If you draw a blank as to what to write, then write, "I want to know what is for my highest good, what would bring me the greatest fulfillment, utilizing my unique talents and expression and bringing me abundance, health, and supportive people and surroundings."

What would bring you the greatest joy? Write asking for your highest or greatest expectations. If you could have the best possible day or week, what would it include? Include spirituality and what your ideal spirit-filled life would be like.

Place your requests in your box. Remind yourself, "My request is being answered. It's in the box. Help is on its way." You might even start singing these phrases. This exercise starts building your trust and belief again.

Personal Letters Go in the Box

Write a personal letter to yourself listing all the things you do well, everything you enjoy about your character, all your accomplishments, and the happiest moments of your life. List all the ways you are grateful.

Write about your appreciation for your willingness to change and learn better ways of using your time, energy, and life. Gratitude for even the smallest everyday things you take for granted is very healing. You may sometimes forget where you've come from, and that you and others have done the best you knew how in any situation. Give yourself and others credit. It is time to heal and embrace your sacred self.

Love Letters Go In The Box

Write a love letter to yourself as if you were your own greatest admirer in a nurturing, healthy, genuine way. God or the Great Creator created you to know and feel that you are special and have a purpose that's rewarding and fulfilling. Begin to spend more time on the good things about yourself and less and less on being a self-critic and indulging body hatred. Treat yourself as your own best friend. How would you like a very special, significant person to treat you? Start there with an attitude of gratitude by writing. Place your letter in your special box.

Place Your Future in the Box

Write your ideal future, about how you want your life to look one to six months from now. If it feels hard to imagine, exaggerate and write it like a fairy tale, allowing yourself to dream of the endless possibilities available to you. If you can see it in your mind, you stand a better chance of creating it. Use a pretty colored piece of paper to remind yourself you are special.

Bless each request and letter before releasing them into the box. Then trust the process.

Keep your goals to yourself; imagine them placed in your heart. Sharing them with others sometimes invites them to be destroyed by the disbelievers through their body language, words, or actions.

Exercise 4 - Sometimes I Need to Talk Loudly!
Use when scared, tense, stiff, and barely breathing.

Create a safe space where you can make as much noise as you want and need. With no one else around to hear, start by breathing deeply and remind yourself that hidden hurts are riding on the breath and being released. Make sure you are comfortable.

This exercise can be intense. I believe we each know our own limits; if you begin to feel too uncomfortable during the exercise, stop. Don't ever force yourself.

Start by talking as loudly as you want, getting your feelings out until you notice your breathing becomes fuller and more from your belly. Voice those negative feelings in a safe environment where you can say all the things you could never say to anyone else. Use your voice; don't damage it, but shout loudly about how badly it feels to hurt so deeply. Cry, wail, yell. Keep going deeper, looking for ways to put sound to your feelings.

Moaning without words is very helpful; use nonsense sounds that express your inner hurt emotions. Wounded spirits moan until words can express the feelings. Or, moan until you feel better, because it doesn't matter if you don't understand why you were stuck or shut down emotionally. This can work, however silly it may appear.

One place to do this is in your car. Park somewhere away from others. Create a special space where you can feel safe just to be yourself without interference from others. When through, open the windows and let the breeze sweep your feelings out into the sky. When they are gone you are one step, or many, closer to freedom. Notice any changes in your breathing, and begin to breathe fuller.

You or others around you might believe that anger, and getting loud, is a sin. However, if anger is disrupting my well-being, I'm ready and willing to choose those exercises that will free me from feelings of "evil" into "live," which are the same letters, only spelled differently. For me personally, sin is only missing the mark and not the damnation and judgment I once believed. Having released this belief that was for me personally damaging, I am able to free myself from the bondage of anger.

You can do the next exercise separately or in conjunction with this one.

Exercise 5 - Laughter Heals
Finding joy, even if it means sounding ridiculous.

Laughter is another tool for recovery that helps us feel outrageously silly and love it. Laughter brings us back to our joy. "A merry heart does good like a medicine," says the Bible. In our pain it's hard to laugh, but some have healed major health challenges by using this exercise. Try it if you care to "laugh with yourself." The first minute or so may seem foolish, but try it; you may even enjoy it. Five minutes later it will be easier; you'll start to laugh at your own jolly sounds.

Choose healthy tools to assist your mind in getting you to laugh; avoid comedy or jokes that degrade others. You can rent or buy comedy videos, CD's, and tapes, or choose to be with a special friend who makes you laugh. Storytellers have delightful stories available in books and tapes, and may even appear in person at local events, covering everything from children's stories to history.

Exercise 6 - Music Uplifts
Changing your mood and feeling better

Music can and will improve your mood. It's hard to stay sad if music is joyous and upbeat. When feeling lonely, disconnected, and empty, take time to find a radio station, cassette, or CD that makes you feel better. Attend a concert, symphony, or opera. Health and happiness go together, so choose to have praise and joyful music fill your soul. It's a great home remedy for getting us out of the blues and into sounds that inspire our bodies. Let your body dance and move to the music. Sing or hum. Soon you'll be breathing freer and feeling more self-love. Be romantic and pretend an angel is dancing with you and you are starting, as of this moment, a new, playful life. Stuffed animals are great helpers; try singing and dancing for or with them.

Caution: if you start feeling lonely, remembering special times in the past, acknowledge the memories, but refocus your mind. This is about creating joy in the moment, not living in the past.

If you are in bed you can imagine dancing. Create costumes to wear and delightful places to travel along with people to meet. Better yet, have a friend tell you uplifting stories.

Books on tape are also available; choose what you would like to feed your mind. Local libraries have motivational tapes and videos on travel and many self-help topics.

Exercise 7 - Creativity, a Key to Healing
Get involved in crafts or hobbies.

Art and creativity lead us back to self-expression and are a key to connecting more with our souls. Go through local newspapers and find meetings to visit or workshops to attend. Enroll in classes at a local center or college. Recreational or activity centers are great sources of classes.

Caution: people recovering from emotional and physical challenges want to look for activities where they can feel safe and welcomed as friends, not treated like strangers. Take time before paying for a class to sit in on a session. If you like it then enroll for a series of classes. If you don't, pay for that class only. Remind yourself that you're looking for a class to help you feel better, and something that is creative and fun. Look for something where you can be involved, and avoid activities that feel boring, stressful, or where you feel out of place. This is a time to reclaim the artistic child within. You may have to push through isolation and shyness, but do it!

Get out and meet supportive people who are doing something to enhance their own self-expression. Life is short! You can start just by making a personal commitment. Many churches or recovery meetings will allow you to barter or attend free if you have no money, so dismiss lack of money as an excuse. Reach out for help. It's waiting for you right now.

Exercise 8 - Making Decisions
What exactly do I want? And how do I feel about it?

You'll need a pad of 8 1/2" by 11" paper. Draw a line down the middle of several pages. On the top left column, write "Things I Like." On the top right column write "Things I Dislike." Choose a subject about which you desire clarity. This may be a personal, career, or health decision. Now write all the things you like about the topic on the left-hand side. In the right column, write all the things you dislike about the topic. Writing faster is better; go beyond the conscious mind into your own inner truth. Don't judge why you feel the way you do. Just vent your dislikes and support your likes.

Review your list. What are the top three to five likes and dislikes? Which column had more writing? Are there obviously more reasons to make one decision than the other? Have the dislikes multiplied, allowing you to see clearly that there is no way this situation will work out?

The result will usually identify itself. If you don't get a direction, wait a day or two and do the exercise again or perhaps reword the question you are asking.

If the conclusion appears to have good points, but you're still feeling some hesitation, then ask yourself: does this represent my integrity, and is it spiritually for my highest good? If the answer is yes, then proceed. If the answer is no, wait, wait, wait. Something better will direct you.

The goal is to move out of fear, doubt, and confusion into more joy and clarity. What would bring you joy? Or support your health and happiness? Choose carefully what represents you very well. Go for first class, not second best.

Exercise 9 - Make Signs
The mind loves to be reminded of what is possible!

* I ask to be delivered to my purpose and passion.
* Show me love today.
* What others think of me is none of my business.
* Life is about being and feeling my divine goodness.
* My job is to take better care of me; God will reward me for my efforts.
* My responsibility is to protect my sacred space and let my good flow into me.
* I'm no longer the prodigal (son or daughter). I've returned home to receive my divine birthright and inheritance.
* I will avoid the three C's: criticizing, condemning, and complaining.
* Gosh, I love myself!
* I'm great, getting greater.
* Prosperity, creativity, and joy go together; I'm guided to experience more of these.
* I'm a precious child of God, special in every way.
* I'm surrounding myself with only those people who are supportive of who I am.
* I love myself the way I am; there is nothing I need to change or rearrange.
* Yes, Yes, Yes!
* I'll fake it until I make it; my life is good now!
* Nothing is more important than feeling good.
* Little flowers always turn to the sun; I will turn my life around also.
* Life is a gift, a gift for living.
* Miracles are happening today.
* Work and play are one.
* As I create in love a product or service, money and every good thing reward me.
* I give God the credit for healing my life—divine timing, not mine.
* I'm succeeding in business and enjoying it.
* God has an image of who I could be with God's traits.
* I'm no longer in denial about my addictions and negative traits; I will do whatever it takes to awaken to my inherent spiritual sacred self in this lifetime.

Exercise 10 - Your Space and Environment
The opportunity to discover stillness and serenity within yourself.

Choosing to stay away from negative situations and people is a powerful way to affirm your worth and create a better and safer future. It's sometimes helpful to treat yourself as if you are in an emergency. Emergencies help us get our priorities straight and treat ourselves with greater respect. If you had no choice but to protect your environment and create a healing space, how would it look and who would be there? Who or what would have to be eliminated or diminished?

Sometimes I wasn't strong enough to tell someone that I couldn't tolerate his or her negativity or that I needed time alone, so I made up a story that my doctor (remember God or Jesus can be your great physician, so you don't have to say who your doctor is) requested that I spend time alone to heal, and I was to rest. I made myself unavailable, choosing whom to talk to and deal with, unplugging the phone at times, or leaving the answering machine to take all my calls. I reserved my time for healthier, more enjoyable people and things to do.

It takes great patience and compassion to believe healing is possible. Pray, believing and reminding yourself often that **"nothing is impossible with God."** Make wise and intelligent use of all the healing agencies available, especially those that nature has so generously placed at your disposal.

Use my story if you need reassurance; it has been a long, long road to recovering and rebuilding my entire body temple. My goal was to create an interior environment of peace; it has been the greatest prescription I could have ever given myself.

PART FOUR
Principles To Live By

I now joy-fully introduce you to principles to live by. Start here as you refine your journey through life. Stay ready and open, knowing through your spirit you will find the potential for all healing and love.

Reflections

My life is like a stained-glass window; many separate pieces make it whole. You'll recognize my stained-glass window, for when the sun comes shining through, rainbows of dancing colors will shine all over you.

May your life be filled with happiness as the sunlight shines within you. We'll journey together sharing Joy-Full stories as the sunlight of God comes shining through.

Blessings. Live your joy.

CHAPTER FIFTEEN

Seven Sacred Self-Improvements

Taking action towards a happier, healthier lifestyle involves the following:

1. **Moving Ahead**
2. **Emotional Healing**
3. **Self-Talk**
4. **Getting Honest**
5. **Self-Love**
6. **Living Spiritually**
7. **Label No Longer**

Read through all seven actions, and pick your favorite to implement for a week or a month. Try journaling your experience and notice months from now the changes that have taken place, and validate yourself.

Practice your chosen self-improvement often to learn a new habit. Be gentle with yourself if you miss a day; just start over fresh the next day. Make every day a new beginning. Expect to be pleasantly surprised.

Exercise 1 - Moving Ahead

Start doing more of what you want, enjoy, and love. If you had plenty of money and were healthy, what would be your heart's desire? Make a list and start (even in a small way) acting as if you already have manifested what is on your list. Before making decisions, you might want to refer to the chapter on "Measure your Joy." If your list falls in the category of numbers six to ten of the Joy Measurement Guide, then proceed.

Create things to look forward to daily, weekly, and monthly. You may decide to plan a trip, start a new hobby, purchase self-help books and tapes, write overdue letters and cards to friends and family, read inspirational books, take dance lessons, make plans to change careers, laugh more, spend more time in nature, and/or schedule emotional or physical therapy.

What you see and hear, you will start believing. Fast from the news for a day or a week; don't listen to the news on radio or TV or read the paper. Notice how you feel and sleep. Take this same time and do something nurturing and healthy for yourself. Break out of automatic routines that aren't life giving.

Exercise 2 - Emotional Healing

Start to honor your feelings more and verbalize your wants and desires. At first it is wise to do this in safe places with people you can trust not to shame you. The rewards include higher energy and increased self-respect. When you stuff or hold back your feelings to please others or feel you are not important, your source of energy diminishes and eventually may cause illness and pain. Stop worrying about hurting or disappointing others if it costs you your emotional health and well-being. Learn to release your emotions as they occur.

Emotions are very real and valid; respect the incredible joy and empowerment that comes from self-expression. It will move you into greater and greater aliveness and health. Get help if needed.

Avoid emotional confusion and indecision; they are paralyzing voids. If you are too confused to make a good decision, get quiet until you can trust your intuition once again (refer to Chapter 14, exercise 8 – "Making Decisions").

Exercise 3 - Self-Talk

Become aware of your self-talk. What do you tell yourself? Would you be proud to tell this to someone else? If people could hear your inner self-talk and see how you treat yourself, would they learn about love and kindness? If not, practice every day by changing your inner language towards yourself and others.

Thoughts held in your mind produce their own kind. Try kindness and compassion! Avoid words of lack and limitation; stop mind gossip of fear and worry.

Start with a segment of time to learn a better way. Perhaps every fifteen minutes, start over. Practice until you develop a habit of utilizing your mind and self-talk to represent your goodness and what you want to attract in your life. Like a magnet, you attract fear or love.

The mind sometimes finds it easier to have negative thoughts than positive. Retraining the thought process takes a willingness and a desire to change, to learn a new habit. It starts with a desire to create a better attitude and healthier results.

Experiment with imagining your inner language being recorded on a cassette tape. You are monitoring the words being recorded, keeping those words that represent the new you. As negative, self-abusive, or non-productive words go through your mind, stop! Stop the mind from grumbling. See yourself cutting the tape, removing the negative words. Splice the tape with imaginary magic glue, restoring and keeping what you would like.

After a day or two the mind will respond to your efforts and your self-talk will get "cleaned up." Because you can't have a positive and negative thought at the same time, choosing better ways to use your mind and sending direct positive messages and impressions to your body eventually affects and attracts a healthier lifestyle.

Exercise 4 - Getting Honest

Be willing to do whatever it takes to shed addictions, compulsive behavior, dysfunction, and negativity. This might include getting therapy, changing your residence or career, making new friends or new relationships, discovering how to play, changing your diet, nurturing yourself, and doing exercise. For some it takes accepting a new way of thinking and living.

Make a list of people who support your goodness, who are positive and uplifting, and call or spend time with them. Start to eliminate those people, places, things, and thoughts that keep you in negative turmoil. Remember the saying: "Let go of the rock if you don't want to drown." Life is meant to be good.

Exercise 5 - Self-Love

Stop starving your body of self-love and appreciation. Recognize and appreciate your body—whatever its size, shape, or condition. Honor and love it as you would a hurting child, and stop all hatred, judgment, and condemnation. Be gentle with yourself. If you hadn't been hurt, there is a big possibility you would never have developed an "I'm not OK attitude," or if you didn't have a need to please others, you would love yourself the way you are with nothing to rearrange or change. Be willing to make improvements but not from deadly self-criticism.

Express your thankfulness daily, even if it feels mechanical at first. Do a personal inventory. Give thanks for your mind and your ability to think. Give thanks for your eyes and your ability to see. Repeat this for each body part; don't miss even individual fingers that serve you every day.

What's inside counts! Get a book on human anatomy and physiology with pictures. No part of the human body works in isolation, yet the owner of the body often forgets to appreciate the beauty and wonder of the interior. Explore, study, and appreciate the reliable gift of your internal "faithful servant."

Create enough special ways to appreciate your body that you notice how much you have to be grateful for. Repeat often, "I've got an attitude of gratitude."

Now appreciate all the support, caregivers, food, housing, clothing, and abundance that serve and surround you. Tell others, "Thank you for making my life easier" or "I really appreciate you."

Exercise 6 - Living Spiritually

Convincing your mind of your divinity and goodness can happen in a brief moment or be one of your greatest challenges. Language and knowledge are quite limiting; learn to depend on your senses to "know for you." It is more a heart-knowing and awakening than doctrine and theology. One can read volumes of books and search various religions and miss the mystical experience in discovering silence, stillness, and serenity.

For some, the messages of being separate from God and not quite measuring up, or being abused or neglected have left deep emotional scars. For some, it takes starting to debate with themselves if separation is really true or not; maybe you have never thought about it much, yet it may be a real breakthrough or turning point, perhaps recognizing the sacred in you for the first time. Perhaps even ask yourself a direct question such as, "If I were God would I cause suffering?" or, "If I were a father or mother would I want my children to be punished through pain, addictions, and dysfunctions?" Decide what you want to believe or not believe, but stop any and all hatred. Choose wisely, because our beliefs do make a difference in our everyday life.

Ask yourself right now, "What would it be like to feel or live more spiritually?" Your heart and soul know the truth: you are part of the universal God presence. You are a precious child of God. Once the truth is recognized and wins the debate, a shift in your body takes place. The shift in consciousness from self-doubt to knowing brings about a shift in the body that is freeing and comforting. Self-love and appreciation start to grow. The internal struggle of feeling empty and lonely starts to cease. You start to realize you are part of a bigger plan; your life has meaning; and, you have a unique purpose that no one else can fulfill.

Growing into greater awareness of your "oneness with God" is not so much a ritual, yet it can be, as much as awakening to the awareness that "you always have been part of the universe and therefore God." Gradually you will stop mistreating yourself, and instead start living with incredible self-respect and integrity. Most of you, my friends, will never, ever want to hurt yourselves or be hurt again.

The truth seeker's biggest heart's desire is to embrace the kinship of God the Creator with you, the created. Love relationships grow from spending time together and from setting up conditions that make love possible. So, how can we begin to acknowledge our Creator?

Contemplation Exercise on Nature

One way to convince and still the mind is to take some part of nature, such as your favorite flower, and spend time with it. Notice each petal, veins in the petals, curves, shapes, and colors. Are the textures rough or smooth? Which do you like best? What intelligence allows it to turn to the sun? (Or what intelligence turns it to the sun?) Could this same intelligence be encouraging you to "turn" and learn a better or healthier way, seeking more sunshine experiences?

Then in the stillness, ask yourself more questions about the creator's characteristics. Describe the life force that created the flower. Where did that force get its education and exquisite imagination?

Observe and look deeply into the heart of the flower. Who could possibly care so much for detailed precision for you to enjoy?

No two flower petals are identical. Why is individuality so important?

Next observe that the creator of the flowers also created you. Go through the questions again; ask similar questions. Who or what created you? Take time to realize that you came into this world with a purpose and talents, unique and individual. No one exactly like you exists in the entire universe. You have great resources available and potential to fulfill your every heart's desire.

Locate chapels, temples, and churches. Go in between services to experience stillness and silence. Visit often. Hundreds of people have prayed and worshiped in these structures. The silence can be overwhelming. It's a real feeling; it's called love. Love heals even when we are unaware of its happening. Over time you will acquire a hunger to experience more of this inner peacefulness. Nature trails and remote locations create this same inner sweetness; embrace your own uniqueness as part of the universe.

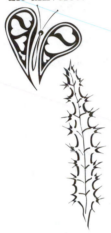

Become as a small child, listening with anticipation for direction and wisdom from inner inspiration. Retreat from the city and relish the opportunity to seek out solitude. While you are there, observe nature. Notice, for instance, the butterflies that seem to know they have a short lifetime, choosing flowers or beauty and color and drinking deeply of delicious sweet nectar to get nourishment. Then fluttering around, they land for just a brief moment on a dried-up, prickly thistle, quickly making a decision not to stay in this uncomfortable, non-life-giving situation.

Many of us have stayed in "dried-up" careers and relationships when it was time for our spirits to go on, but we stayed sitting on the "thistle." Eventually we experienced pain and discomfort, and some of us had to almost lose our joyful-spirits before we would let go. Many more of us are no longer willing to settle for the "thistles" in life, but instead choose the "flowers," creating more joyful experiences with passion and purpose.

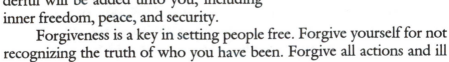

As your love relationship for God, nature, and yourself grows, so will your spiritual gifts, and your purpose will become more obvious. All things good and wonderful will be added unto you, including inner freedom, peace, and security.

Forgiveness is a key in setting people free. Forgive yourself for not recognizing the truth of who you have been. Forgive all actions and ill feelings towards yourself and others. This can be done in person, in writing, or in a ritual of releasing the past.

"We've all done the best we knew how." Forgiveness forgives even if it appears impossible to forget. **"I realize you must have been really hurt in your life to ever pass that hurt onto me. I know no one would ever hurt another if they hadn't already been damaged. For your actions and patterns I forgive you."** I know all people are created to love and be loving towards themselves and others. We can change by loving ourselves and set an example for others.

Let this greater love be shown in your living and working space by creating beauty and order. Strive to replace the old stuff that no longer serves your new awareness. Create a sacred space for your sacred self.

Exercise 7 - Label No Longer

Don't accept a negative diagnosis or opinion from anyone. Even today, doctors claim that rosacea cannot be cured, only controlled with medications; yet I was healed. You and the Creator who created you are in charge. Seek out people who are into choices, and those who can work with you in affirming your goodness. It might mean treating yourself like you are in an emergency, letting go of what is not working regardless of the price or effort it takes, and placing you in top priority.

Keep your focus on the healthy parts of your body. For example, if five percent of your body has an illness or disease, then focus on the ninety-five percent that is healthy. Send love, not fear to that hurting five percent. Take time to love the pain. This may be difficult to do when pain hits, but even small ways are helpful and noticeable. Let it tell you its story; it is trying to get your attention. Treat that part with kindness, nurturing, and high respect, not resentment. It is possible that it will redirect your life in a positive way.

If you are making a transition through death, it doesn't mean a healing isn't taking place. Healing emotionally, physically, mentally, and spiritually transforms you to your next experience.

CHAPTER SIXTEEN

SEEK WITH PURPOSE AND PASSION

Seek God's Free Physicians

Fresh Air
Pure Water
Sunshine
Exercise
Rest
Power of the Mind
Imagination
Prayer

Seek God's Natural Healing Process

Acknowledge your physiological body responses.
Learn to release your emotional feelings
Heal your emotional pain and negative memories from the past

Seek God's Masterpiece

Learn to be proud of your unique characteristics, weaknesses, and strengths

Seek God's Joy

Your Purpose and Passion in Life

Seek God's Attributes

Integrity
Honesty
Truth
Faith
Hope
Love
Peace
Joy
Discernment

Seek With Purpose and Passion

Seek God's Harmony
Create Harmony and Beauty

Seek God's Natural Garden
Eat plenty of vegetables, fruits, seeds, nuts, and herbs.
Eat a variety of whole grains and beans.
Drink pure, fresh water.

Seek God, Your Creator
Create conditions and time for the opportunity.

Seek God's Artwork
Enjoy sunsets, the moon, flowers, babies, animals, rivers, and other
wonders of nature.

Seek God's Abundance
The world is full of possibilities.
Plant an idea, nurture it with love, watch it grow, and reap its
bountiful blessings.

Seek Reasons to Give
Share your talents by giving the overflow of the love you feel toward
yourself to others.

Seek Forgiveness
See unloving actions, about yourself and others, as convoluted ways of
asking for love.

Seek Wisdom
Be nonjudgemental, for you see others through your own eyes.
Seek and see only good; it will reflect who you are.

Seek Trusting
Believe that only good is happening despite appearances.
The greatest rainbows follow the worst storms.

Seek to Keep on Seeking
Being more JOY-FULL

Index

A

abundance 37, 85, 86, 106, 118
accomplishments 28, 36, 37, 106
addiction(s)
      3, 15, 31, 34, 35, 36, 42, 59, 60, 74, 85, 86, 99, 101,
      111, 117, 118
alive 11, 20, 28, 37, 44, 45, 50, 95, 106
angel 105, 106
anger 15, 21, 25, 31, 35, 36, 58, 61, 62, 85, 88, 104, 105, 108
angry 9, 10, 16, 31, 33, 35, 56, 87, 88, 98, 102, 104, 105
arthritis 7, 17, 32
aura 63

B

balance 8, 13, 61, 62, 63, 76, 78, 79, 81, 97
beauty 7, 37, 42, 43, 44, 69, 100, 118, 120, 121
belief
      14, 31, 34, 35, 36, 38, 41, 60, 93, 106, 108
belief system 5, 22, 25, 27, 105
Bible 21, 37, 108
blood 4, 7, 26, 41, 55, 97
blood sugar 72
body memories 24, 25, 26, 27, 28, 59, 101, 102
bread 7
business 3, 6, 8, 15, 18, 20, 36, 40, 41, 42, 46, 111

C

church 16, 17, 18, 21, 22, 35, 36, 37, 47
cigarettes 16, 74
colon 6, 76, 77, 78, 81
colonics 6, 28, 77, 81
compassion 17, 34, 38, 45, 47, 82, 90, 96, 112, 116
confusion 22, 23, 35, 41, 55, 110, 116
creativity 24, 34, 36, 56, 57, 96, 111
Creator 21, 35, 104, 107, 119, 121

D

dance 27, 70, 116

freedom 16, 27, 34, 63, 64, 108, 120
fruit 6, 7, 14, 21, 71, 72, 77, 99
future 4, 37, 45, 50, 51, 65, 78, 92, 94, 95, 96, 99, 102, 107, 112

G

garlic 7, 11
God
  3, 7, 9, 10, 16, 17, 18, 22, 23, 25, 34, 35, 36, 37, 38, 40,
  41, 42, 43, 44, 47, 49, 53, 55, 60, 63, 64, 65, 81, 82, 83,
  86, 92, 93, 97, 100, 102, 104, 105, 107, 111, 112, 118,
  119, 120
God Box 105
grateful 10, 50, 57, 106, 118
gratitude 19, 20, 23, 36, 40, 44, 107, 118
grief 9, 31, 33, 62
guidance 5, 22, 24, 40, 45, 55, 59, 63, 64, 83, 106

H

happiness 14, 56, 57, 60, 63, 83, 95, 101, 104, 110
harmony 7, 13, 14, 24, 28, 42, 50, 60, 62, 79, 80, 100

heal
  6, 8, 11, 12, 14, 15, 16, 21, 23, 24, 25, 26, 27, 28, 29, 30,
  36, 37, 43, 47, 48, 49, 50, 51, 62, 69, 74, 81, 82, 91, 95,
  96, 97, 101, 103, 104, 107, 108, 110, 112, 120, 121
healing
  4, 7, 8, 10, 11, 12, 13, 14, 15, 16, 19, 20, 21, 23, 24, 25,
  26, 27, 28, 29, 30, 31, 34, 35, 37, 39, 41, 43, 45, 47, 48,
  49, 50, 57, 58, 60, 61, 62, 63, 64, 78, 79, 80, 81, 82, 87, 89,
  92, 93, 96, 97, 101, 102, 103, 104, 107, 111, 112, 115, 116,
  121
health
  3, 7, 8, 9, 11, 12, 13, 19, 21, 28, 29, 31, 36, 40, 42, 45,
  50, 57, 60, 61, 63, 70, 71, 74, 77, 78, 81, 82, 83, 90, 96,
  101, 104, 106, 108, 116
health food store(s) 6, 71, 73, 77, 78, 80, 82
healthy
  5, 13, 14, 28, 30, 37, 38, 43, 56, 60, 61, 64, 65, 73, 74, 77,
  78, 88, 90, 93, 94, 95, 96, 97, 101, 103, 104, 107, 108,
  115, 116, 121
herbs 7, 31, 82
history 30, 31, 36, 39, 44, 92, 93, 94, 95, 109
hobby 115
holistic 6, 7, 10, 11, 17, 29, 31, 80, 81, 82, 101

129

Share the Joy!

Order additional copies of Joy-Full Holistic Remedies for:

Family and Friends
Co-Workers
Support Groups (use as a study guide)
Book Stores and Libraries
Spiritual Growth Groups
Holistic Practitioners and Teachers
Gifts

For quantity discounts, please contact us.
We have T-shirts, too!
Order one of the two logo styles shown below:

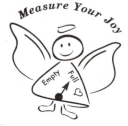

Item JF

Item MYJ

To order, visit our web site (www.joy-full.com) or use the convenient mail order form provided on the next page.

We invite you to share with us how this book has helped you or someone you care about.

Write or E-Mail:

Joy-Full Publishing Company
P.O. Box 591661
Houston, Texas 77259-1661
joy_full@earthlink.net

JOY-FULL MAIL ORDER FORM
Complete and return to address listed on previous page.
ORDER FIVE BOOKS AND GET A FREE POSTER!

	Quantity	Total
Joy-Full Holistic Remedies Book $12.95 ea.	_____	_____

Purple Cotton T-Shirts/White Logo
   Item #JF "Joy-Full Holistic Remedies"
   Please indicate S, M, L, XL _____   _____   _____
   Item #MYJ "Measure Your Joy"
   Please indicate S, M, L, XL _____   _____   _____

Poster: "Seek With Purpose and Passion" - Chapter 16 text $4.00 ea.
Purple print on white card stock, 8 1/2 X 14   _____   _____

   Subtotal: _____
   Texas residents add 8.25% sales tax   _____
   Shipping and Handling (see chart below)   _____
      Grand Total   _____

If a gift, how would you like the card to read?_____
_____

Shipping and Handling
0 - $12.00   Free   Alaska, Canada, & Hawaii
$12.01 - 12.95 3.50   add additional $3.00.
$12.96 - 30.00 4.50
$30.01 - 55.00 5.00   For international orders,
$55.01 - 80.00 7.00   please contact us.
$80.01 -$125.00$10.00
$125.01+ $15.00   Allow 3-4 weeks for delivery.

Shipping Address (PLEASE PRINT):

Name_____
Street Address_____
P.O. Box (if applicable)_____
City_____State_____Zip_____
Home Phone_____Work Phone_____

Please make checks payable to Joy-Full Publishing Company (U.S. $ only)

CREDIT CARD INFORMATION   Visa____   MC____
Name as it appears on card (PLEASE PRINT):_____
Credit Card Number_____
Expiration Date_____
Signature_____

Prices subject to change without notice.